WE Danced

OUR STORY OF LOVE AND DEMENTIA

SCOTT M. ROSE

WE
Danced

OUR STORY OF LOVE
AND DEMENTIA

Dedication

For those who have danced.
For those who have loved and laughed.
For those who have sought their true selves.
And for those who have lost all they cherished most.

Maureen's Journal – 2/27/97

*"I have no idea why God made me the way
That I am, but I am thankful he has brought
Such happiness and contentment to my life,
And, of course, the laughter."*

Contents

Preface

*M*aureen Patrick-Rose warmed hearts with her gentle smile until her passing October 10, 2019. Her spirit softly touched so many lives but always in a simple, understated way. Unless of course she knew you well; then laughter and gaiety ensued. Her life, love, and sickness warranted telling grand stories as both inspiration and life lessons. Her nature, though, would command nothing more than a heartfelt nod of remembrance on a special holiday. That nature made her all the more beautiful and her story all the more worth telling.

She never let life make her cynical. She remained hopeful and grateful. She saw the wonder in things, whether big or small. She delighted in the spectacles of Niagara Falls and the Grand Canyon as well as the simple pleasures of a single rose in her garden or a field of tulips. She would chase whales off the Kauai coast and stand silently gazing at a hummingbird among her Fuchsia. Maureen cherished the brush strokes of Monet and rode a bicycle through the French countryside. She relished coffee chats with old friends and rocking her firstborn grandson as he slept. She saw the beauty in all things. She allowed herself to be amazed. She allowed herself to feel the awe of it all.

Maureen's diagnosis with Frontotemporal Degeneration (FTD) in June of 2016 shattered our world. It left us stunned. We never realized how profoundly that disease would integrate with our lives, until of course it did.

Dementia does not change a person fundamentally, which I know will have many up in arms in disagreement. It presents tremendous challenges, no doubt. It changed how we approached our days, but no disease could break our deep love or what we meant to each other. Even when dementia-fueled fits of anger swept over Maureen, I knew I had to help her and wait it out. The love of my life remained inside her somewhere. Even when she could no longer translate into words, "This is my husband," she knew me still. She knew me to be safe, comfortable, and someone she could trust. She knew I cared for her deeply. For me, that was enough.

In writing this memoir, I struggled with the question of when Maureen's story should start. I could go back to her birth, April 27, 1950, or further back to her mother or father's childhoods, as their lives certainly shaped hers. As I am her third husband, perhaps I should only go so far back as when I first met her—June 28, 1993. While I had no intention of writing a book about Maureen at that time, I saw a person struggling to find her voice and respect and justice under extreme duress. Those feelings certainly shaped aspects of the story contained within these pages.

I could begin with July 22, 2000, when she shared with me tremendously personal revelations of pain and struggle and love with such a fierce timidity, yet so vulnerable to me alone. All the facets of her personality that I knew so intimately before came together then. All that I knew of her paled in comparison to what I saw in her then. I wished everyone had known the strength of this often shy and introverted woman. I married her a little over four months later.

However, I think the final push that made me write this book really came much later. Life's daily crises tend to push our dreams and passions out a bit longer than intended. Weeks become months become years. You devote yourself to a person, very willingly, and thoughts of publishing a book seem like such far-off fantasies. They recede into the background compared to the importance of spending every available moment with the love of your life. Maureen too dreamed of writing a book, so this book is as much hers as mine.

I think on the number of journals that we started and stopped. We scribbled entries not much longer than the love notes we would trade. Our spontaneous and vivid lives did not fit neatly into some heirloom tomb. We expressed them so openly and regularly with "I love you banana bunches" Post-its near the coffee maker.

I think the book idea really started shortly after October 22, 2018, when a closed social media support group under the umbrella of the Association for Frontotemporal Degeneration (www.theaftd.org) accepted me in. Before all this happened, I had almost no experience with dementia. I had never even heard of FTD. After Maureen's diagnosis, I read. I read a lot. Online searches would bring up these support groups that I dismissed as distractions from caring for my wife. However, the more she deteriorated, the harder the care became, and the more I realized nobody around me either could, or would, help. It became apparent a support group might boost me up in my down times and guide my endeavors.

Men often have a hard time admitting they need a support group—one of the true tragedies in modern society. Men think they must do things on their own, that they just need to "man up", and that needing help signifies weakness or failure. Thank God I did not hold to that belief system. I still retreat to my cave from time to time to work things out, as the male brainwashing runs deep, but this group made such a difference.

I read many of the posts in the group from caregivers with loved ones suffering with FTD. It surprised me to also see posts from those actually suffering with the disease themselves. I followed their stories, and I would share vignettes of our life with FTD. I walked that fine line one travels between maintaining your wife's privacy and sharing the graphic details for her betterment and others'. I hope that I did not cross that line.

Most of the stories that I read in the group poured out from caregivers understandably full of anxiety, sorrow, and despair. For them, this sounding board allowed them to wail and receive comfort and understanding from those that truly knew. For some reason, I approached it differently. I wanted to inspire. Do not ask me why, I just had some deep-seated desire to be the helper guy or knight in shining armor—a persona that my wife had indulged me in for nearly two decades.

I started to become recognized as a regular poster sharing stories of humor, tenderness, and hope. I kept my intentional humor self-deprecating—but never at the expense of my wife. The love and inspired language just sort of flowed with it. I held tightly, every day, to my hopeless love for my wife—I was "smitten", as I would say. I refused to give up on her and kept looking for the rainbows among the ruins. I would spin a positive out of something as simple as me changing her shoes when she would have them on the wrong feet. I tried to show that we all struggle. Let us address it, move on, and find the next happy moment rather than wallow in the idea that this happened for the third time today.

Accidentally grabbing your fork for soup does not define you or your loved one. Our character, our hearts, and the breadth of how we live our lives better define us than a single errant decision on any given day.

I tried to bring that kind of thinking to the support group. I found later that some would eagerly await my posts. I would receive private messages when I had not posted in a few days, "I just want to make sure you are ok. I haven't seen a post from you this week, and I always check for them on Sundays."

I encouraged others to "celebrate the magnificence of the ordinary," though I found Maureen anything but. My growing collection of stories caused several readers to suggest compiling them into a book. While many might have instead started a blog, I wanted to share a larger story to a wider audience. The story went beyond the AFTD postings. Our love story, well before FTD of course, held an equally important role for me. The story of Maureen herself resonates for me as more important than the rest.

The biggest inspiration proved to be my love for my wife, her story, and all that she embodied. That story of her, and of us, shaped how we tackled FTD together. No doubt our approach differed from others'. But I cherish this journey of ours as both beautiful and flawed. I invite you to mine your own nuggets from our lessons—not just in dementia, but in love.

I found a note in my phone from 2/26/19: "Book Title—We Danced: Our Story of Love and Dementia," so I guess that notion held through today.

Scott M. Rose
Portland, Oregon
Spring 2021

Acknowledgements

I think on the people most supportive of our story and of Maureen; they made this book happen. That support in troubled times allowed Maureen to continue to spread joy and love and to receive it. That support made our love story possible.

Her dearest friends Candy, Jeanne, Esther, Cindi, Fernie, Margo, and Dawna gave her joy throughout so much of her life and influenced so many stories in this book, so I thank you.

Thank you to Lauren and the Association for Frontotemporal Degeneration (www.theaftd.org) for providing a safe and supportive space to share aspects of our journey together.

The appreciation I feel would not be complete without recognizing those people that shared their support for me through our personal journeys together in FTD. Those direct and intimate conversations made me realize the importance of sharing this story. Thank you, Amy, Lauren, Melissa, Brendan, Tom, and Steven.

My lifelong friends checked in to make sure that I could manage my grief and provided support for me in big and small ways. Charles and Cam, Angela, and Allison I thank you.

Thank you to Parkview Memory Care and Northwest Hospice that tirelessly provided Maureen's care in her last fourteen months and practiced an ongoing commitment to better understand FTD.

To the Pittock Mansion Society and the Portland Parks Department, thank you for assisting me in creating a memorial to honor Maureen. It brings me comfort when I feel at my worst.

Never forgotten, thank you to the many caregivers and loved ones suffering with FTD that post their journeys regularly for us to receive and learn from. May we find inspiration to give generously of our resources and time to support education, awareness, and research for a cure.

As my wife remains the beginning and end for me, the inspiration for all that I have achieved and ever will, I offer my eternal appreciation to Maureen. You remain the love of my life, my baby, my everything. I hope I do justice to this piece of your story.

Introduction

We hear of the trials of marriage. Dementia adds another facet to that struggle. I call it a struggle, but Maureen and I never really struggled with marriage. Sure, we had rocks in the road, but as our favorite pastor once said, "There are two kinds of people: those who stop and stare at the rock and those who just go around it."

How you approach life certainly dictates how you approach marriage and, unsurprisingly, how you approach sickness.

In my proposal to Maureen on September 1, 2000, I quoted *Song of Solomon*, "You are all fair, my love, and there is no spot in you." I saw her as perfect and asked her to marry me as proof.

We marry "in sickness and in health"—never more tried than when your beloved has dementia. In this book, I will explore the ravages of dementia on Maureen and how we overcame it to keep our marriage strong 'till the moment I held her hand and watched her breathe her last. To this day, I have never experienced anything so painful. You will think that you prepared yourself. I will walk you through the steps, but that will not matter when you find yourself in the middle of it. Your whole life crashes in front of you.

I have attended no less than one hundred seminars and presentations related to my career and have presented on similar topics twice as many times. The repeatable theme of the importance of communication comes up so often that it sounds cliché. I would find myself tuning it out the moment they went down that familiar rabbit hole. Of course, everyone needs good communication skills. However, I never want to reduce my wife to a talking point. I find her story worth telling in all ways and in all places, no matter the context.

Have you ever stopped to think about how you communicate? Do you really communicate well? How do you know? Do you have frequent misunderstandings, frustrations, silent treatments, or shouting matches? If so, I would argue that you do not communicate well.

A marriage involves multiple ways of communicating. We employed all of these in our marriage and pushed the limits with the dementia. Because of our closeness, we did not even know when we did it.

Now imagine the further complication that dementia adds by taking away your ability to reason or interpret things correctly, or to use familiar words, and as such hamstringing your communication. Imagine that frustration for someone to think one thing and know they said something completely different but cannot control it. Imagine you have lost the ability to write or to read or to even point at a picture board to indicate what you want. Now you have a picture of the language side of FTD. Now, imagine you, as the caregiver, on the other end of that trying to serve your loved one and not having a clue what they want to communicate. How do you overcome this?

You start to see another aspect of the challenge. You start to see the dance.

My wife had Frontotemporal Degeneration. The medical industry characterizes FTD as a progressive disorder of the brain effecting language, behavior, and/or movement. The industry also refers to it as Frontotemporal Lobar Degeneration or Pick's Disease. My wife had semantic variant Primary Progressive Aphasia (svPPA), one of multiple clinical subtypes of FTD:

Behavioral Variant
Primary Progressive Aphasia (language) Variants:
    Semantic
    Agrammatic (nonfluent)
    Logopenic
Movement Disorders:
    Corticobasal syndrome
    Progressive supranuclear palsy
    FTD with Parkinsonism
    FTD with amyotrophic lateral sclerosis (FTD-ALS or FTD with motor neuron disease).

The commonality between the subtypes of FTD? As of this writing, there is no cure and it's fatal.

As I stated, my wife had the svPPA.

She started out with difficulty finding the right words and losing the understanding of what certain words meant. She would talk about things in vague terms, often dropping nouns, using similar sounding words, or even confusing pronouns. Her struggle to sort things in her head, like her birthday, came across as memory loss. She did not have memory loss.

Obviously, when you see yourself struggling with these things, you speak less and do not want to communicate, because it feels impossible.

She had difficulty understanding what other people said, especially when receiving and acting on instructions. Whether someone provided new instructions or her brain was incorrectly telling her how to use familiar and typical objects in the home, it developed into an immense struggle. It quickly escalated to the point that she would freeze—unable to proceed. She developed problems with reading and writing, eventually to the point that she could hardly do either. Imagine having full use of your hand but being unable to tell it to sign your name.

As the disease progressed, other symptoms developed: changes in her behavior, senses, and mobility.

The preparation I offer in this book more illustrates how we responded when that storm came. If you take pieces of it to weather your own storm, all the better.

I struggled with categorizing this work. Is it a memoir or a romance? An instruction manual or a self-help book? Is it a collection of poetry or a journal/blog hybrid? The fractured method of telling this story and sharing lessons learned both in love and sickness represents the varied materials that I drew from.

I offer everything honestly from reading our journals and my firsthand experiences. I think of author John Pavlovitz, who said about losing a dear loved one, "You lose the part of you that only they knew. You lose some of your story."

That intimacy of our story binds the glory and tragedy of romance. Maureen and I would share countless tender conversations, revelations, and the undying devotional whispers of two people so desperately in love. These occurred almost anywhere: in a bookstore, sitting at a gas station or in a car wash, walking in the park, or repairing a dishwasher. Love remains constant, and the lovelorn do not let changing a flat tire get in the way of expressing, "You are simply the best thing to ever happen to me." True story!

So many of my wife's accounts of her life started with some fear or trepidation on her part that would cause me to momentarily stop the world from turning. I would place one of her hands between both of mine and assure her, "It's ok baby." She would respond, "I've never told anyone this but…", and then share another facet of her life from before we were us.

She never made up stories or sought to draw attention to herself. Maureen never had a motive of gain in recounting any of these events. As such, I have no reason to doubt them.

This sharing partially defined our early relationship. At first, these revelations seemed like her method for letting me know what I had gotten myself into and to allow me to bail on the whole affair if I chose (I never did, save once, to my shame). After we married though, they came about out of utter trust. She knew that nothing she shared could shake what we had. On this point, I could not have agreed more.

These random anecdotes from her life confound my grasp, like gathering bits of confetti and trying to sort them back into a whole. My memory captured the most significant aspects, however, many of the finer details I have pulled from love notes, partial journals, emails, holiday cards, social media posts, books with notes in the margins, Post-its, and handcrafted mementos with our sweet nothings scribbled along the edges.

The fractured sources and format of this book align quite elegantly with its divided purpose. Maureen lived beautifully—with grace and kindness. This story primarily revolves around her: the broken but strong woman, quick to love, slow to anger, quiet and misunderstood, yet kind and dispensing joy with an unmatched heart. This story also chronicles her three and a half years of FTD. I recount the progression of her dementia through, and including, her passing and our strategies to withstand it. I hope that it can serve as a collection of recognizable guideposts should you find yourself in a similar situation.

Above all, our story tells of love—simply love.

Love causes us to rejoice, to bloom, to peak, and to transcend. It also exposes us to our greatest sorrows, pain, and a longing that simply goes unfulfilled. Loving someone comes simply. However, holding onto that love reveals its countless facets. Life works to shatter as many of those as it can. We employ stories to keep it together—keeping those shards from shattering on the floor.

Stories themselves, however, require action too. Nobody ever gained worthy trust through words alone. Love takes a lifetime of action—turning words into reality.

While Alzheimer's ranks as the most common form of dementia, FTD ranks as the most common form of dementia for people under sixty. That makes this a critical story.

Why should you read this story? I offer two reasons. First, FTD remains one of the most devastating diseases in the world and one of the most misdiagnosed. The more you know, the more you can offer compassion and understanding.

Second, I provide you with our love story. Love affects us all.

Chapter 1

Maureen

"*I*'d brush my dolls nearly bald."

Maureen loved hair her whole life, whether her own, a friend's, her doll's, or the movie stars with lives in the faraway places that she dreamed of.

She grew up in central Oregon in the small town of Redmond with her parents and older brother...and her calico cat Tiger. Her brother had a Lab, but Maureen had little interest in the big dog as it bounced up on everyone and "made a mess," as she put it.

Maureen preferred quieter things. While she would play with neighborhood kids and join their outdoor games like Kick the Can, Annie Annie Over, and Hide-and-Seek, or ride make-believe horses in the canyon, she also spent a lot of time alone or one-on-one with a close girlfriend. They would brush their dolls' hair and imagine them on great adventures. Maureen also loved to read—whether the classics or comic books. She had a bookcase with a sliding door built into her bed's headboard—perfect for storing books, gum, and treasures.

They lived in a two-story home with her and her brother's bedrooms upstairs and her parents on the main floor. They painted her bedroom walls lavender, and she had flowered drapes and a white cotton bedspread.

Her older brother enjoyed arguing with Maureen, simply for the sake of arguing. He would take an absurd position, just to argue. They fought. While she loved her older brother, she also resented the double standard of what he did around the house compared to her. He had a single chore: to take out the garbage. After school, he would grab a Coke and chips and camp out in front of the TV. Her father also liked watching television in the late evening, preferring Milton Berle and *Gunsmoke* and followed later by *Bonanza* and *The Flintstones*.

Her father leased a butcher's shop in the Piggly Wiggly grocery store. He bought and cut the meat and marketed the shop. Maureen's mother greeted customers and helped with the books. Maureen comically developed a dislike for lamb. For whatever reason, lamb rarely sold. Her father would bring home the meat about to turn so as to minimize losses. That meant a lot of lamb! Maureen would start hiding it in her napkin after a while.

Maureen was very close to both her parents, but in different ways. Maureen's father treasured family and especially doted on Maureen. He quit smoking shortly after the war, so he always had toothpicks and lifesavers in the breast pocket of his starched white, short-sleeved shirts. Maureen would greet her father at night and steal a lifesaver and a kiss.

Her father, full Irish, had given Maureen her name after the actress, Maureen O'Hara. He also chose her middle name, LaVaye, shrouded in mystery as something he brought back from his time in France during World War II. Her mother often shortened it to 'Reen, or Maureen LaVaye when she was in trouble.

Maureen had more of a structured relationship with her mother. They loved each other for certain, but chores, etiquette, and expectations better defined their interactions. From early on, Maureen had a long list of chores to do around the house. Her mother made lists every day.

Maureen made her bed and cleaned her room as most kids did. However, she also washed and folded clothes every day and started to cook the dinner and set the table before her mother got home. Dinner was not 'till 8 p.m. She washed the dishes every night and maybe got to read a little after. Every weekend, every inch of the house was cleaned in terms of dusting, floors, changing sheets, and laundry. She ironed pillowcases on Sunday nights, as well as hand-kerchiefs and scarves. She grew to hate ironing.

There was little time left for play or fun. Maureen would tell you she had a good life, but a lonely one with very few close friends. Candy was one of her earliest and closest friends. Maureen would recount much later in life, "Candy and I have been best friends and like sisters since we were five. Candy is one of a kind—a kind, generous, and gracious person who always sees the positive in everything. She has been such a giving person in my life. She is the one person I can always rely on. We have shared the good and bad times, and not once did she fail to be my friend. Never. I love her like the sister I never had."

Sadly, Candy moved away when they were nine, so they had to keep in touch with letters and very few visits. While some friends remained, Maureen often felt lonely and isolated.

The family remained in Oregon throughout Maureen's child-hood, save for the three-hundred-mile summer trek to Weiser, Idaho, where Maureen was born and where her mother's family still resided. She loved her grandma and grandpa on her mother's side. Her grandma would let Maureen use the vanity and brush her hair with the mother-of-pearl comb, brush, and matching hand mirror. She would also let Maureen help in the flower garden, sit at the old writing desk, and play at the large piano in the parlor.

Her grandmother also made them go to church, though Maureen did not really mind, as she liked the songs and had a good head for memorizing some of the prayers.

Her grandfather and uncle would saddle up their respective horses for real riding adventures; much more satisfying than the pretend horses in the canyon back home. Maureen also helped with the cows and collected eggs. Her grandfather let her do just about anything, including sitting in the yard eating the tomatoes and cucumbers or playing in the hay before bringing it over for the horses. She would skim the cream off the milk in the mornings for her cereal.

They would also visit her father's family. Her father's mother was bright, but strict and not as open. That grandfather was a dark and disturbed man, and he molested Maureen at a very young age. Sadly, they did not talk about this behavior in the fifties, and left Maureen to feel she had done something wrong, as she had nobody to talk to about it. This trauma served as a foundation to Maureen's lack of confidence and self-worth and later intimacy issues.

While the early years were a financial struggle, Maureen defined them as middle class and comfortable. At Christmas, they would decorate big. The aroma of candies and cookies would fill the house, as would the fresh juniper and evergreen. They would always have a tree, and on some occasions her father would flock it—ruining more than one vacuum in the process. Each year, Maureen would stare at the lights on the tree and front of the house, captivated. Even her usually bothersome brother really shined at Christmas, helping with the decorations and doing his most to give nice gifts to everyone. Maureen would always receive nice gifts, including her first Barbie—what hair!

She and a friend imagined all the things their dolls would do, places they would go, and clothes they would wear. Their Barbies were actresses or cheerleaders or secretaries—such were the expectations of the time.

Maureen lived close to her schools, so she mostly walked, though she sometimes took the bus during the harsh winters with its snow, ice, and the wickedly cold wind. She would wear leggings under the dresses her mother made her wear. She wore rubber galoshes on those walks and changed into other shoes at school.

Maureen started playing the alto sax in the fifth grade, so she had daily practice requirements on top of her homework and household chores. While she appreciated the opportunity, she gravitated toward the small family piano every chance she got. Her father could play it by ear, and it always excited Maureen to listen to him play.

At this same time, she had trouble seeing the blackboard and was prescribed glasses. "I felt ugly and hated them. I also started changing physically, and I felt uncomfortable with that because no other girls were changing yet, and the boys were making fun of me. Mom never talked about such things. It seemed as if these subjects were forbidden."

Her mother would put her in lovely dresses and get her hair styled in just such a way—pretty but at the same time so formal, like a doll, that it made her an easy target for teasing. Her mother once cut her hair into something between a bob and a bouffant. Maureen simply yearned to let her hair grow long and wear it in a ponytail like her friends. She lived through the growing sock-hop craze of the fifties. She saw Audrey Hepburn and Brigette Bardot in the movies and thought, "Yes, like that." She combed the curls right out of Barbie's "out-of-the-box" bouffant. She considered it as her silent protest to her own hair.

Although Maureen had several lovely dresses, she feared she looked more like a doll than a girl who would PLAY with dolls, or listen to music, or talk about silly girly things. Her friends started wearing pedal pushers, pleated skirts, and bolero jackets with scalloped edges—even cotton overalls.

Maureen had a hard time expressing her hopes as a child. Her words often came across as unpardonable sass. She loved her mother dearly but hated the lack of control over her own life and choices. She had many chores from the moment she got home from school to "keep her out of trouble." Years later, some of her lifelong girlfriends still recalled Maureen's strict schedule. She was being groomed as the perfect housewife. She knew it and hated it.

Among these emotional trials, there were also expectations for social gatherings and clubs. Her mother pushed the family into higher society to help them climb the social ladder (wanting to leave the poor life of Idaho behind) by joining the bowling team, helping with the March of Dimes dances, becoming members of the Elks and the 75 Club, and hosting Pinochle parties. She placed the pre-teen equivalent expectations on Maureen, which proved troubling for such a reserved and self-aware girl, but she tried.

Her parents would host socials at home sometimes. Maureen would watch from a dark corner and sometimes disappear into her mother's room, where she would slip on her mother's petticoats and heels. She would drape her mother's rabbit stole over her shoulders. She would play with the lipstick, eye shadow, and nail polish. She would put on her mother's gloves and cart her handbags around in the quiet comfort of a private room and away from prying eyes. She would hear the music and bustle in the front room and pretend she was at a ball. In private it was ok, but in public, she panicked.

On other nights, after all her chores were done, Maureen would quietly go to her room and pull out a book. By the sixth grade, she had been introduced to *Beautiful Joe* and lost herself in the wonderful story. One year, she asked for a date stamp for Christmas. She lined up all her books and would play librarian until her mother called up to go to bed and turn off the light.

As a teenager, Maureen continued having issues with her image. She moved away from more formal dresses and started wearing stretch pants and miniskirts with mohair or Angora sweaters. She still wore glasses 'till she was sixteen, when she pleaded for contact lenses. She had severe teenage acne. Mealtime was torture. The family rules required that everyone take two helpings, which caused Maureen to gain a lot of weight. These issues all lead to more bullying and caused Maureen to withdraw to only her very closest friends.

At her mother's urging, she joined the Pep Club and the Honor Society as part of the expected social norm. Her mother pushed her into society though Maureen felt completely unprepared and could not talk to her mother about her anxiety.

Maureen got jobs babysitting and filing invoices at the meat market. She eventually got a waitressing job. She started in the back washing dishes until she grew in confidence and started waiting tables out front. She had a great memory for orders and was very polite to the customers. In the summer, they served the firefighting smoke jumpers. On one occasion, Maureen brought six such men split pea soup and spilled it all over one man's lap. She fled to the back and remained there all night—mortified.

At home, the attempts to make her more well-rounded, more social, and more fitting as a future wife backfired to some degree. They worked, but she hated it. When I say she hated it, I mean she hated playing a role that someone else had planned for her. Her dreams held no value. She could not discuss them.

The family did not take vacations for the most part. Maureen did enjoy the summer trips back to Idaho to see family and day trips to the local lake to water ski. They took one flight to Florida her senior year to see her father's relocated brother. Other than that, her boundaries were fixed in Oregon and Idaho, but Maureen longed to see more. She wanted to see the faraway places that she read about or heard about from others. Some of her parents' wealthier acquaintances would tell stories of other states, countries, and continents, and the exotic things they saw there.

One would never describe Maureen as lazy, unappreciative, or spoiled. She had dreams. She dreamed of having worth and someone respecting her opinion. She wanted a voice rather than being on display as a reflection of her parents or future husband. Her dreams remained private hopes. Her lack of self-confidence kept them silenced.

Maureen always returned to her hair to express herself—her ONE rebellion. As a teenager, she wore her mother down and eventually got to wear her hair long. She would straighten her blond locks with an iron.

The success she had in controlling her hair blossomed into confidence in those late teen years. She had a couple of girlfriends she would drive with to the local A&W to buy Cokes. She went to dances with her parents and eventually to school dances as well. She got over her awkward stage and started dating cautiously.

Maureen did well in school (she was fifteenth in her class) and received awards in science and music, including an invitation to play the saxophone at a state competition. She loved to write as well. She looked forward to the day that she could go to college.

Her older brother enrolled in the University of Oregon. However, when Maureen graduated high school, her parents denied her that same opportunity, even though she had received a partial scholarship. She pleaded her case, but as a woman in the sixties, she lost that battle.

Instead, her parents sent Maureen to Merritt-Davis for nine months—a small business school in rural Medford that taught secretarial skills. She received her certificate, returned home, and quickly married her high school sweetheart. She had learned to keep a home, and he had a traditional family, so her domestic training suited everyone fine.

Maureen loved her first husband and did desire marriage, children, and a home of her own. But she also wanted to matter in her own right for her thoughts and ideas. Life quickly beat that dream down. She came to concede that most people measured a woman's worth in how she ran a home and in her service to her family. As such, she realigned her dreams. As money was tight after they first got married, they both had to work odd jobs. Two children followed quickly. They remained always in Oregon, living in Bend and Portland briefly before settling in Eugene.

Maureen saw her husband as a good man. She also saw that he looked at marriage very differently—likely just a product of the time. He brooded over odd jobs and working indoors. He loved camping, fishing, and boating. But having limited funds, he did not see much of that. When an opportunity opened up to work with a river guide, he jumped on it. That type of seasonal work meant Maureen had to make up the difference best she could while running the household. Things seemed flush in the summer but lean the rest of the year. She worked to save money and canned their vegetables, but with her husband's growing outdoor business, he needed more equipment. This often burned through their modest savings.

These growing needs sometimes put them at odds. Her husband wrecked and then sold Maureen's car that her parents had given her for graduation (a 1968 Firebird). He sold her grandmother's piano too. He sold both without asking Maureen. She simply found them gone one day. This broke her heart. She came to justify it as being for the business and, as such, for the family. She mulled over her bigger sorrow that he never asked if he could sell those things—her things. The money she would save for the house would go missing as he would buy guns and hunting dogs and was always trading for different trucks. She had no say in any of these purchases, and it wore heavily on her.

Her mother and father divorced a few years after Maureen got married. She had seen them growing further and further apart, and Maureen tried to play both sides of the fence.

She loved her mother and understood why she had left. They had many conversations about her personal struggles and her father's temper and night screams—leftovers from the war. Her mother made a new life with a job in Eugene and would soon remarry.

Maureen also spent time with her father. The divorce and the fracturing of the family placed him into a depression. Her older brother had married and moved away as well, so her father saw it all falling apart. He treasured family and had passed those values on to Maureen. He cried on Maureen's shoulder several times. He later married a woman in town. With new regulations forcing him to close his butcher shop, he took up the insurance business, though he never felt at peace with it. Maureen understood that and spoke with her father about it. He also got his real estate license, which appealed to Maureen as one of her own dreams. But he never got to use it.

Through his depression, he did little and gained a lot of weight. He became irritable, except toward Maureen, with whom he maintained a close relationship. He had forgone most outdoor activities when his brother Lowell asked him to go out on a hike in the gorge. Out of shape, he had no business saying yes. Maureen's father died from a heart attack on that trip in 1975. Lowell blamed himself for years. Maureen sobbed, and to some degree, she never stopped missing her father.

With her father gone, her brother married and moved outside of Portland, and her mother now remarried and often on trucking routes to California with Maureen's stepfather, Maureen felt alone. As such, she refocused on her own family.

Maureen had two children, a daughter and then a son. She loved life as a mom. She would always save a little money that nobody else knew about to make sure the kids had good clothes and presents at birthdays and Christmas. The kids made her cards for the holidays, especially Valentine's, and she loved and saved them all. She worked a job, maintained the house, and then worked her second job for the river guide business. Her husband had at least two complete sets of gear. He would come home and drop his gear, pick up the other, and leave again. Maureen would get the gear cleaned, restocked, and ready for the next trip. Sometimes with larger groups, she would come along to set up and strike campsites.

Oddly, for a river guide, her husband did not like people much. However, no people, no job. Maureen's requests to go up to Portland at Christmas time or to see distant family and friends were always met with resistance. When they did go, he would last only a short while and then retreat to the car or shuffle them off as quickly as they got there. During a couple of reunions (more like large camping trips) it seemed tolerable. Maureen would plead for a little more time but would lose most of those battles.

She would maintain her friendship with Candy through long spells of not seeing each other. Candy had married a good man too, and they had two children very close in age to Maureen's two. The families would occasionally go camping together. While always a lot of work, they enjoyed it and did it whenever they could. However, even just going up to Vancouver, WA to visit, Maureen's husband resisted hard. That, or he would remain angry the whole time and drive them back as soon as possible. He started to drink a lot, and it became embarrassing for Maureen. Any time she would mention it, he would immediately get mad. She longed for travel and real vacations but could see that she dreamed those dreams alone.

Her father had left her a small inheritance—not enough to change their lifestyle, but Maureen put it away into savings for a future house. Sadly, when it came time and she advocated for a particular home, her husband dictated another. The four of them moved into a home with several problems, but like so many things in her life, her opinion simply did not matter.

Over the years, they settled into a routine: Maureen raised the kids and maintained the house and worked. She eventually got a job with the school district transportation department driving school buses so as to get on similar hours as the kids. Her husband continued the hunting and river guiding. He would rarely agree to come to the kids' activities or sports and grew more distant. He would come home from a trip angry and leave angry, and Maureen just felt like she could not win.

In the early eighties, Maureen started to bargain with God to try and turn her marriage around. She went with a neighbor girlfriend to get baptized and then asked God to heal her marriage. Surprisingly, her husband came home early from a trip that night. They talked for hours, and she told herself that God had helped them turn a corner. It did not last a month.

Maureen thought she had driven a permanent wedge between them when she held her ground with a couple of things she saw as wrong. Her husband would meet all sorts of different people as a river guide. Some he would connect with outside of the trip. A few wanted to come over to the house with drugs. Much later in life, Maureen recalled that it took all her willpower to muster the confidence to insist, "No." She said they could not bring drugs into the house with her kids. Her fear at that moment left her shaking. Her husband stood by, furious and embarrassed.

On another occasion, a couple from one of the rafting trips asked them if they wanted to swing. Maureen flushed, the rage and shame from her childhood abuse flaring up. She threw them out. Again, the wedge deepened between her and her husband. She curled up in a ball and cried alone at the thought of what they had asked. She became resentful that her husband had even placed her in that position.

It took great effort for Maureen to feel good about herself, and some people in her life took advantage of that. Maureen wanted to see the good in everyone, sometimes at great cost to herself. Very few people in her life felt toxic enough to cut off completely. She did not hesitate to cut off people who were bad for her children. But to cut off people who were bad for herself, she had to first muster the self-confidence and realization that she deserved something better. That, each time, became a much longer journey.

Understanding that they had grown apart over time, Maureen tried to start anew with her husband by arranging date nights. These went poorly. He did not want to go out. He preferred drinking, puttering in the garage, and putting together his gear.

Maureen recounted one such date night, when she had had enough. She had given her husband several days' notice that she wanted to go out to a movie, just the two of them. Maureen had found the movie time and arranged the babysitter. They did not have a lot of money, so she made dinner at home. They would go to the movie after. She made Reubens while he puttered in the garage. She waited and waited, reminding him a couple times of the movie's start time. She finally brought one of the grilled Reubens out to the garage and set it on his work bench next to him.

She walked away and asked him to please hurry, as the sitter had arrived and they had to leave for the movie soon. He said nothing. She turned at the doorway and asked him if he had heard her.

He glared at her, took the plate, and dumped the sandwich in the garbage. She held her plate with her Reuben on it, grabbed the hot sandwich, and threw it at him. It hit him right on the side of the face. Years later she would laugh about this, saying she had no idea how she aimed that so perfectly. She slammed the garage door and sent the sitter home.

These vignettes illustrate their life—two separate lives. Her husband wanted their eventual retirement to consist of travelling the local skeet-shooting circuit. Nothing could have been further from Maureen's hopes and dreams. With her kids now teenagers and into their own things, Maureen felt alone and vulnerable. Her mother was always on the road with her stepfather, so she was seldom nearby. Maureen had made a few friends in the neighborhood, but her best lifelong friends all lived in other towns. From there, things went from bad to worse.

Maureen drove school buses in Eugene. She knew the area well, and people knew her as a very competent driver who could take any route. She felt she had some value there. She knew how to control the kids on her bus too. They stayed in line, though middle schoolers often proved the biggest challenge. On one occasion, they would not settle down, so she threatened to stop the bus 'till they did. Ignoring the warning, the kids continued. She pulled the bus over, took out a book, and began reading. When the shocked kids realized they could not get home, they settled down. She looked back in the mirror, saw angels, put the book away, started the bus, and continued. She grinned each time she told that story.

Recognizing Maureen for her good work, her supervisors promoted her and moved her from driving to dispatch (still with the occasional relief driving). She took to it flawlessly. Once, they even asked her to speak to the department about a new routing program. While flattered, she found it terribly nerve-wracking and clumsily stumbled through it. Her lack of self-confidence remained a lifelong struggle despite the fact that others found her very capable, personable, and intelligent.

Her direct supervisor in dispatch often complimented her on her work. Unfortunately, he too had marital problems. The cliché of complaining about your marriage to someone of the opposite sex at work who also had marital problems had not yet become a cliché. They got too close. Maureen saw someone who openly praised her, who talked of travel, and who seemed to listen to and understand her. She saw an opportunity to perhaps realize some dreams. After all, her mother had left a relationship that no longer worked and appeared much happier. Perhaps, she thought, she should too.

Maureen announced she was leaving at her daughter's graduation party, but her supervisor did not follow through with leaving his wife as he had said he would. Maureen, in her hopes for a happier and more fulfilling life, had made a series of bad choices. In reaching for a way out, in an instant, almost everyone around her labelled her a slut and a homewrecker. Devastated, she cried about the choices she had made.

Maureen moved into an apartment with her two kids and managed the divorce from her first husband. While furious, he also refused to find a balance between their home life and his river work. Maureen knew their relationship had deteriorated beyond repair, even before the infidelity. She regretted hurting him and apologized. He hurt her too but refused to acknowledge it. Sadly, because of the way she handled it, nobody cared to hear her side. She found herself sinking further into sadness and despair from all the talk she heard from every direction.

Of course, her supervisor's wife soon threw him out of his house, so he couch surfed a bit, even staying at Maureen's apartment with her kids. They eventually got married at a civil service performed by his uncle, a judge. They bought a home together with a bedroom for his young son, whom he had partial visiting rights to.

The house included rooms for her two kids as well. However, her daughter had moved out and into the home of a boyfriend's parents. Upset with Maureen, her daughter had little to say to her. But then her daughter's situation with her boyfriend blew up, and she called Maureen to bail her out. Maureen of course helped her daughter move out and had her live with her—no questions asked. Maureen also later took in, for a few months, one of her daughter's friends who had a hard home life of her own. Maureen had a big heart. That girl remained thankful to Maureen for the rest of their lives.

Maureen's son wanted to live with his mom, but he did not like her new husband. Instead, he moved in with his dad. That did not last and had its own share of problems. He wanted to move back in with his mom. The back and forth broke Maureen's heart. She sat her son down and explained that her house had no revolving door. She welcomed him with open arms to live with her, but he could not keep moving in and out, as it hurt too much.

Maureen patched a family together as best she could but did not see the slow transformation taking place. Her new husband did not warm to her kids and actively tried to recreate his prior family. He convinced Maureen to cut her hair short and dye it red. Both he and his young son were redheads, and he thought they needed to look like a family. Desperate to make it work, she did not see the manipulation...or denied it. Her new husband, like her first, also drank. He drank a lot. At first, Maureen convinced herself that he did it to cope with his recent losses and the upheaval in his life.

Then, she suddenly lost her job in his department.

They shuffled her off due to a rule that married couples could not work in the same office. Maureen became the one to move, the one to start over, the one to continue under duress and with imposed shame.

They sent her to an administrative position in a relatively new department in the district. They called it the Capital Improvements Program (CIP). This was where I first met Maureen.

Chapter 2

Wonderful Friendship

The CIP Department managed capital school construction projects for the general obligation bond passed by the Eugene School District. It paid for capital improvements at all the schools. I had worked for the Feds in the General Services Administration office in Portland, Oregon a couple of years, where I finished my degree. With that position dissolved and the job market generally poor in 1989, I went to the Seattle area and worked for the Kent School District in their Capital Projects Department. After four years there, I missed Oregon and looked for an opportunity to go back. When Eugene passed their bond and advertised for project managers with school experience, I applied. They brought me in as the third of four project managers and I started work there in May of 1993.

At twenty-six and building my career, I got in at the ground level of this program. They needed driven, committed managers. Each of us would have a high school region with some overlap between us. I liked the fast pace, but unfortunately it also came with long hours. We figured out protocols and practices on the fly from each of our past experiences. We had one accounting person and one administrative person for millions of dollars in capital work. That proved too great of a challenge. We needed another administrator. The district found us one from Transportation. They advised us that this person came from the Transportation Department because of a forced move due to rules in place regarding married couples in the same office. She had office experience but was new to anything regarding facilities and would need coaching.

The two project managers first hired had developed a good rapport with the current administrator, so another manager and I would get this new person and would need to break her in and show her the ropes.

I remember the day Maureen arrived. In an admittedly tough job, she already came in beaten down and self-conscious. I saw her visibly nervous. I saw someone who did not want to be there. I only understood later that they had given her two choices: take this job or leave the district. Naïve to politics, and not much interested in them either, I simply wanted an administrator to help with the load and was happy to receive one. The quicker I could make her feel at ease and bring her into the processes, the better.

We welcomed her aboard. She received some basic orientation from the other two ladies in the department. I waited until the latter part of that first day and then introduced myself one-on-one. I told her about myself and asked about her. Maureen smiled, but she had a lot of walls up. I asked whether she had any kids, and that eased her tension. She liked to talk about her kids. I then asked her what she knew about our department. Not much! I thought to myself, "How do you just drop someone into this kind of job with no guidance?"

I did a download of what I knew and then asked her what she wanted from her role. I remember her answer vividly, "I honestly don't know. I am supposed to help in the office. I am supposed to help the project managers."

We spent a few days together outlining each of the projects and establishing a list of duties. It all seemed detached to her, like things just floating out there with no semblance of meaning. I saw in her a smart and capable person, no doubt. I tried to make it about projects and not people, as I sensed trust would take a while. She had a lot thrown at her. She brought a light lunch each day, hardly anything. She sat at her desk with a book. Sometimes she would leave on a walk alone at lunch or sit on the fire escape.

In this new department, project managers were in charge of hiring the architects and builders and served as the liaisons to the teachers, principals, and other technical staff to make sure the construction scope was aligned with the educational and physical needs, the budget was met, and the schedule was maintained. In the summer, school renovations and construction move quickly, with lots of details to work through, and I and the other project managers ran all over the district putting out "fires". Maureen's primary tasks were to make sure contract documents and communications continued to flow between all parties while I was out inspecting the work at job sites. We would circle back with each other multiple times per day so she did not feel like she was diving into the deep end. While out, I found a deli in my work region that worked for a quick go-to lunch. Occasionally, I asked Maureen if she wanted me to bring her back something. She always answered, "No."

After a few weeks, it seemed like Maureen didn't really talk to anyone else aside from the one other administrator and me. She still seemed sad, but perhaps no longer miserable. I saw that as progress.

Several consultants and contractors would work on any one project. I could see it was all just names and numbers to Maureen. She sometimes got projects confused. I suggested that she come with me to the job site meetings for a few weeks to meet the people in the field and associate names with faces and tasks. I thought that would also give her a stronger sense of construction projects.

The internet had not caught on big yet, and we had just started using email. That sped up correspondence and expectations. We had the big brick phones, but reliability remained spotty. I remember the day in early August when it all seemed to click for Maureen. A small issue came up that I would normally review, but I had other challenges outside of the office. The email came in, and she remembered hearing about it in a job meeting that I had taken her to. Because of that knowledge, she could respond to the question. She sent an answer off and resolved the problem. I came back in the office and heard what happened. She beamed, like it had all just come together. Maureen had turned a corner.

From there, she gained some confidence. She went into the field with me more and walked the sites to see the construction firsthand. She took on more work from other managers as she got work done at a faster pace. She did good work, too. She let her guard down a bit and started chatting with staff in the building from the other departments. She let me bring her soup from the deli on occasion. By fall, she had become one of the team.

She also found someone in me that she could talk to about art, music, movies, and old books. I had a passion for those things too and brought in flyers from the art galleries that I would go to. She was fascinated by some of the art, like Isaac Maimon's café scenes. Most of the pictures were of women sitting having coffee with big hats and colorful hosiery—feminine and playful, seemingly without a care in the world.

Other pieces we would both laugh at as a little too "out there" for our tastes. This all helped to break the ice and increase her comfort in the role she found herself in.

I got back into theater with a couple of productions in town. Maureen wanted to hear about my rehearsals, as she had always wanted to try acting but lacked the confidence and support.

I joined a local poetry group and told her about that. She desperately wanted to do more writing than she had done to date. She then told me about her education and how she would like to take classes. I encouraged her to do so. She let that inspire her to take a creative writing class at the local community college. She aced it, though not without a lot of trepidation. She felt so accomplished.

After that first year, the rumors started. Some staff voiced their concern that Maureen would leave the office to go to the job sites. They asked why they did not get to go to job sites too, or they wanted Maureen in the office more. Some of the managers would go along with this and others not. It created a division. People also thought Maureen and I had gotten too chummy. We would stand talking about our respective weekends on Mondays. The talk started getting back to her, and she resented it. We spoke about it.

"I know people are saying things about me leaving the office and saying things about us. I don't want to care, but I have to. I like what I am doing. I like working with you. You teach me a lot. You didn't care about the baggage I brought here. I like talking with you about art and old books. I don't want to give this up. I'm happier."

I told her I understood but suggested that we adjust the outings to only once a week instead of several days. "Let's get in a regular, predictable pattern. You go to the Wednesday meetings only. Let's slow down on the soups too," I said, "That's my fault."

I did not want to put her in a difficult position, and she did not want to go backwards either.

We adjusted and still maintained a strong friendship, leaving our banter and catching up for the Wednesdays to and from the job sites. It worked, and the talk lessened though it never went away. After the second year, things took another turn.

I burned out. I was working 60-hour weeks, working most Saturdays and the occasional Sunday to keep up with projects. I also came to realize that when I left the Seattle area two years prior because I missed Oregon, I was actually missing Portland. I found

Eugene too small. I also thought about becoming an architect. I had a bachelor's with an emphasis on architecture and urban planning. I was twenty-eight, and if I ever wanted to work as an architect for a firm, I needed to make the leap.

I applied for one position, and they turned me down. I did not have the skillsets they advertised. A month later, that same firm called me back. They had a different position that they thought I would fit perfectly. They invited me up to Portland, interviewed me, and made me an offer right there. That Thursday offer involved a start date of the next Monday.

I told Maureen first, as she was my closest friend. She had a hard time with it. She knew that the job made me unhappy but could not help but think about what this move would mean for her role. Nobody else took her to job sites. Nobody else explained things to her. I had become more than a co-worker, but also a close friend. I told her that I felt the same. I also reminded her that after two years, she no longer needed things explained. She had a wealth of knowledge and would do well. Her confidence remained tenuous but intact. Maureen's confidence always needed bolstering. She had forty-five years of being told her opinion did not matter, and "do as you're told."

Given the short notice, I worked both jobs for three weeks to ease the transition. While packing my things to move to an apartment in Portland, Maureen called me at home and asked if she could come over.

I lived in an apartment building in Eugene that developers had converted from an old school. It had an old gymnasium in the center that they converted into an open-air courtyard with balconies lining it. The wood floors of the old school halls remained. The building had two entries: the old main school entry and the old upstage area of the performance space. They converted the old principal's office into the same for the site manager, and they renovated all the classrooms into one-bedroom and studio apartments.

Maureen arrived holding a small, wrapped gift as a going-away present. We sat down, and I opened it. She gave me a book of poetry; Whitman. I had mentioned seeing it in a bookstore near a place that we lunched at once. She also gave me a journal. She liked the way I wrote. To her surprise, I had a gift for her too. I had planned to give it to her for her birthday a few months prior but, worried about the message it might send to others, I held on to it instead. She had mentioned some beautiful glass wind chimes in a small shop in Bandon, Oregon on the coast. I had gone there to find them and wrapped them up, but then never gave them to her. Now, it seemed like the right time. She cried softly.

We hugged. We had a closer friendship than any other that either of us had at the moment. Her friends lived in other towns or states and kept busy with their lives. I had spent so much time on my career, I had not slowed down to make true, lasting friends. We hugged for a long time. Then she got up to leave and asked me to email her to keep her up to date on my life. I promised. She walked away.

Life and propriety interrupt the best intentions. We wrote periodically, but we kept our emails very matter-of-fact so she could focus on what she needed to at home and work. We wrote about the events and activities in our lives, including my adjusting to the new job and Portland living. She tried to keep her job interesting but had managers that did not trust her to do what she had done for me. She felt her role had gone from an assistant project manager (albeit a role we created together) to simply clerical. It left a void in her work life. For propriety, she did not share all of this with me at the time—nor sadly with anyone else. Her life became darker. She went through what she called her Black Winter.

She behaved oddly around friends, even ones that she had known since childhood. She carried a lot of shame over the last several years of her life and the choices she had made. The guilt built up inside her again. She felt isolation, loss, anxiety attacks, and a lot of tears. She described it in her journal as being "like death".

Her second husband continued to drink a lot and would pass out in front of company. She became so embarrassed and tired of apologizing for him that she just stopped inviting people over. Once, she started making a recipe and could not find the cooking sherry, only to discover that he had drunk it.

His talk of travel resulted in only two trips. They took one up to his uncle's home near Seattle for a small family reunion. The other trip consisted of a weeklong cruise, which he spent drinking most of the time.

Maureen wanted to leave him that winter of 95/96, but she physically and mentally felt she did not have the strength. She felt isolated, alone, and embarrassed. Admittedly though, these feelings did not stem from him entirely but from her own actions as well.

She rededicated herself to making the marriage work, but she did not see him making an equal commitment. He didn't listen to the humiliation she had gone through with work. He showed no effort to try and relate to her children. Her friends and family knew the answers before she did. She sat too close—in the middle of the storm.

She had multiple barriers in her life, physically and emotionally. These prevented her from connecting with friends and family. Her daughter got married. Her son moved out on his own. Her few neighbor friends moved away. She felt alone...again.

Maureen sought the help of a psychiatrist to guide her through this period and to aid her in opening up about her repressed feelings. Maureen found her insightful. This woman helped Maureen see that she had value and, in fact, could think of herself as a good person. The psychiatrist convinced her that she deserved to take some time to heal herself and reconnect with family and friends.

Maureen took a trip on her own to Florida to visit her uncle Lowell, whose wife had contracted Alzheimer's. Their daughter Margo (Maureen's cousin and close friend) joined as well. They thoroughly enjoyed their time together. However, Maureen could also see the toll the dementia had taken on her aunt. She had no idea of the foreshadowing. Related by marriage, this would not impact her hereditarily, but nonetheless, it hung heavily on Maureen as her first real exposure to dementia.

Upon her return, two things pulled her through that spring: church and the birth of her first grandson.

At church, she found peace and acceptance.

Maureen's letter to her childhood friend Jeanne - 6/17/96

"There I felt a calming of spirit and I started working myself back to daylight once again."

She said she kept searching for answers as to why she behaved and thought the way that she did. Her husband rarely went to church, so she went alone.

In April of 1996, her daughter gave birth to her first grandson— just three days after Maureen's own birthday.

Maureen's Journal – 5/7/96

"When I hold you, you are so content and calm. You lay in my arms as I rock and hold you in awe of what a wonder you are. I can't take my eyes off of you for very long."

Maureen's same letter to Jeanne - 6/17/96

"I have the most beautiful grandson God could have ever sent me. He is my salvation. When I get lonely, I go and sing to him. He loves the way I sing because I am so enthusiastic."

Her first grandchild was a blessing in Maureen's life. He gave her such joy. She had felt so very low and was in a dark place, but now she relished in this little miracle. The sad reality that Maureen's husband and her daughter did not get along (she had strong trust concerns) just meant that Maureen made more trips over to see her daughter and new family than vice versa. Maureen understood.

Having finished a couple of classes, she purchased herself a journal and began writing and chronicling her time with her grandson.

She also started reconnecting with friends. They had frank conversations. Her friend Cindi had probably spent the most time with Maureen and her first husband in the early years of their marriage. Cindi knew of the good times and the bad. Cindi said she completely understood why Maureen had left her first husband, given the drinking, the lifestyle, and the troubles. She also knew she could now be honest with Maureen and told her that she had left the wrong way. The way she did it caused damage to her relationship with her kids. Maureen appreciated the talk and restoring her friendship with Cindi.

Maureen's Journal – 7/1/96

"I hope Cindi and I are able to continue this healing process. I need these people in my life."

Maureen felt hurt for years but also knew she had hurt others: both husbands, her kids, her friends, and family. She felt the importance of mending those relationships. She knew she had to initiate it.

Maureen and her son had lunch together weekly and talked about that very thing. He said he understood, and Maureen watched her son grow before her eyes. He spoke of taking responsibility for his own life. They spoke not as mother and son, but as two adults. He did not judge his mother. They quickly got past their issues and became very close.

The trust with her daughter proved harder to win back. Maureen spoke to her and apologized for the way she had handled things but also explained that she could never go back to her father, "I am so incredibly sorry for what I did, but I can never again live with your father. The problems are still there with the drinking, the lifestyle, being taken for granted, and the intimidation. I need laughter, fulfillment, and time with all my friends and family. I need to express myself through writing and who knows what else."

At least she had put it out there. Her daughter's new husband had a large family, so Maureen often got marginalized. She understood the healing would take longer with her daughter, but Maureen spent most of the rest of her life making up for what she had done. The relationship eventually mended, but it was never as close as she craved. That saddened Maureen for many years after.

These talks helped with her healing but did not stop the downward spiral of her second marriage. She knew what she had to do.

Her second husband's drinking had increased. Multiple discussions regarding his alcoholism and asking him to seek help went unanswered. She asked him to go to marriage counseling, but he refused to see a problem. His brother also occasionally made drugs available to him. This worsened his behavior. Maureen saw this as a second dead end. Her two children had grown up and created their own lives. Her work became unfulfilling. Her husband drank almost every night and passed out in his chair in front of the TV. He isolated himself from her.

Maureen had had enough of seeing her life stalling. She had gone to church and prayed for answers. She said she felt God nudging her to take charge of her life and latch onto the good things. She decided to leave her husband.

She found an apartment through a friend and reached out to her mother and her son for help. Labor Day weekend, her husband told Maureen that he planned to go to his brother's house all three days. She said nothing and let him go. The moving truck arrived a few hours later. They grabbed everything that Maureen had owned before the marriage as well as a modest amount of furniture. She did not take more than her share and left him with everything he needed.

She took enough to start her life again. "Again," she thought. "How many times do I get?"

They had just grabbed what they thought reasonable. Some things got left behind in a storage closet or cupboard, which she only realized later. They had just packed the essentials and went.

The movers and some family moved her into her new apartment and helped her arrange her things. They accomplished a lot that day. It takes a lot to start someone's life over!

She had left her husband a note in the house explaining everything. She knew he would not take it well, although she also didn't think that he would be that surprised. In her note she wrote that divorce papers would be sent to him in the next couple of weeks.

Her mother, stepfather, and son with his girlfriend hugged her and left. She sat alone in her apartment, staring at the life she now had in front of her. She knew she would not stay alone. She had her son, her daughter, her son-in-law, and her darling little grandson nearby. Now a bit closer to all of them, she could see them more often. She knew she had God in her life too. She knew all of this but had a good cry anyway.

That night she asked God to show her what she should do. She asked Him to put the people in her life that He wanted for her. She asked Him to take away the people that brought her down or took her down the wrong path.

Alone, she thought of me. She asked God to either put me in her life or take me away. A month later, I called her for a business trip.

Chapter 3

A New Start

A year into my new job, I had made strides as someone they could just let loose to get work done. I had an aptitude for client relations and for taking on new challenges. I could present to potential clients and learned the up-front assessment and planning work done ahead of projects. I never got on a good glide path to becoming an architect, and in truth never became one. Instead, they recognized me as a project manager that people wanted on their teams. The bosses wanted to see me on more front-end work. As such, a marketing opportunity arose.

This well-established national school design firm had only had an office in the Oregon market for two years. They wanted to expand their local connections with more districts in the state. They decided Lane County had good potential for work and wanted to do a sweep. The boss remembered I had worked in Lane County, specifically Eugene, and asked me to set something up with my old contacts.

I called the district and got ahold of the administrator who worked alongside Maureen. I let her know of our interest and arranged a meeting with the director for the following week. Late that afternoon, I received a call at the office. It was Maureen. She had heard that I planned to come down the next week. We caught up a bit, as we had not written for a couple of months. She said,

"Before you come down next week, you should know something. I left my husband last month."

The clueless male chip in my brain kicked in, and I said, "Oh, I'm sorry to hear that."

"I just didn't want you to be surprised if you heard that while you were down here," she said.

As fate would have it, my boss cancelled the trip down there due to a bigger opportunity and a schedule conflict. He asked me to let the districts know and reschedule.

I called, and this time got Maureen. "Hi. Hey, our marketing trip got cancelled. I will need to reschedule for another time."

"Oh, that's too bad," she replied, "I was looking forward to seeing you. Maybe we could exchange home numbers and keep in touch."

We did, and we did.

We spoke on the phone multiple times for three months. She shared with me all about her new life. She now watched her new grandson as her daughter and son-in-law worked for a cleaning business at night. They needed an evening babysitter. Her son had a serious girlfriend whom Maureen really liked. Maureen also started going to church regularly, writing in her journal, and joined a women's choir. This all sounded delightfully out of the norm for her. I could hear the happiness in her voice, and I encouraged her. She had not sung publicly since the sixth grade. She said, "I pity those women around me that have to listen to my singing, but it is fun." I knew her to sing beautifully, despite her modesty.

After that three months, I took some time off for the Christmas break and suggested I come down and we go out for dinner. She liked that idea. I drove the two hours down. I got there, said hello, and the dam broke. She gave me a huge hug, and we stood there in her doorway for a long time. I had never had someone greet me so caringly and lovingly, nor had I realized just how much I missed her.

We did not go out for dinner. We ordered Chinese delivery and lingered inside, talking for hours. We had so much more than friendship now. I had never felt anything like that before, and she had not felt it in years, maybe ever herself.

I had Christmas obligations at my family's, as did she, but I offered to see her the following weekend and take her up to Portland. She loved the idea. In Portland I took her everywhere. She wanted to see the shops and streets and Christmas decorations that still remained. They had one Starbucks in Eugene but many in Portland. She loved Starbucks and wanted to go there every morning. She liked the environment and the vibe, not just the coffee. It reminded her of the Maimon art we had both gravitated toward. The atmosphere inspired her to sit and be herself and talk with good friends or someone even more dear. She would tell me for years that she just liked spending time with me.

We also went on our first actual date and saw the movie *Jerry Maguire.* Just like that week before, "You had me at hello." Springsteen's *Secret Garden* remained one of our favorite songs the rest of our lives.

Maureen's Journal – 12/31/96

"Innocent, honest, open, loving, sincere, happy, carefree, serious, and curious. That is the way I want to be with you. Scott, I will always need to know. I will always need to tease so I can see your eyes light up. I will always need to hold and be held. I will always need to gently kiss you, feel you, love you, laugh with you, and talk and walk with you. I want to be the other part of you. I want to help you with your endeavors in life. I want to be your inspiration to

We engaged in a long-distance relationship—new territory for both of us. Two hours separated our homes. I saw her every weekend, either spending it down there or she would drive up. Often, I would drive down Friday afternoon, pick her up to drive her back to Portland, just to then drive her back down Sunday evening. This increased our time together—even just driving and talking. It always made her sad when she had to leave me and drive home alone.

When I drove her back home, I would spend that Sunday night too and then get up before the crack of dawn to drive back to work Monday morning. We would cheat it more with a regular Wednesday job site meeting I would have near her. Yes, we now had our Wednesdays back, similar to before. This time they meant so much more. I would come down Tuesday night and/or leave Thursday morning (brutal, like those early Monday mornings) just to maximize our time together.

We were not the kind of couple to hurry a goodbye.

When I stayed down there, we would often stay in and just make dinner together. I thought the whole relationship would end abruptly one night as I cooked some green beans and dropped a dollop of butter in the pot. She looked at me like I had lost my mind but laughed at the same moment. She had never put butter on her beans. We would laugh about that moment for years. Apparently, some things that I watched my mother do while growing up did not apply universally.

I noticed something as we were together: she chewed several times before swallowing—anything really. She told me she had a small throat and a lifelong fear of choking. In retrospect, she likely chewed as much as my mother asked me to. I just never paid attention. I tried to eat more slowly, but I always seemed to finish far ahead of Maureen. I could see that made her feel self-conscious. I started to talk more during the meal (something my father had always frowned upon) about things we could do, whether music festivals, art walks, or outdoor markets. This allowed us to finish about the same time and grow closer as well.

Fortunately, she found herself utterly in love, and it was the same for me. I would catch myself staring at her thinking about my luck. She had a slender form and stood about five foot five. While she would occasionally dye her hair with some highlights, it hung long, blonde, and straight. She loved her long straight hair and told me how she used an iron to straighten it in her late teen years to make it look like Crystal Gayle or Cher (though blonde). She would often ask me to brush her hair.

Maureen once told me, "There are few things on this earth more intimate or enjoyable than getting your hair brushed."

She introduced me to so much. She had all this nutritional knowledge about whole grains, spices, and vitamins—not just good for you but essential. She often thumbed her book, *Prescription for Nutritional Healing*, like the grail of eating and living. She lived, mostly, the healthier lifestyle. She told me about the nine-inch plates (smaller plates) that people used to eat on. "Over time, plates got bigger and so did waistlines," she explained. She introduced me to a neighborhood bakery that used the best and most wholesome ingredients. She journaled of her dreams to open a natural foods store or café.

She read voraciously. She copied information from books and clipped articles from magazines and newspapers on everything from essential oils to new art exhibits at the university to the benefits of certain plants and herbs. She felt free to seek out the information she had always heard whispers of but never had the support to pursue. Excitedly, she would share all this new information with me over our meals together.

Sometimes our dinner rendezvous would get moved so she could spend time with her kids and grandson. She kept trying to forge new and stronger relationships with them. I understood the importance of that.

I listened to her sing in her women's choir. I went to the church she attended. She would sing there too where we sat together in our seats. However, she loved to come up to Portland with all the things to do and see compared to the smaller venue of Eugene. We saw live music and went to eclectic restaurants: some good and some not so good.

We spoke on the phone a lot at night. I mean for hours, like kids. With this being back in the days of paying for long distance calls, I felt concerned after the first month and thought our phone calls might be costing her a lot. I mailed her twenty dollars to help with her phone bill (we saw each other every week, but who does not like to get mail?). She laughed because her phone bill came the same day. The twenty dollars did not even begin to cover it. I had never made so many long-distance calls, so I had no idea how much it might cost. When my bill came, I understood. Wow! She kept that twenty-dollar bill in her journal for years.

That year, she connected with her good friends near Portland: Candy, Jeanne, Mary, and Dawna. Each had a husband and kids—some kids at home but most grown and gone. She connected with cousins she had lost contact with. She reveled in how alive and happy she felt. She told each friend how she had turned a corner. She smiled so freely, living the life she wanted. She felt she had found someone that valued, respected, and loved her. She had.

Maureen's Journal – 3/10/97

You and I have such a unique relationship, one that borders on all I have asked for. I am finally able to say I love you; I believe in you; you are nice inside and out. I see the same things you possess as you see in me. You bring me to the beauty of words and meaning. You bring me the encouragement to be creative. You are teaching me that I can dream all the impossible dreams and attain them. You show me all the beauty that lies at my fingertips. You show me how to slow down my pace and see, hear, taste, smell, and touch. How wonderful you are. Yet, you love my need to know more, to run, to laugh, to cry, to love, to walk and talk. You love it when I am excited by something new. My whole face lights up, from the sparkle in my eye, to the smile on my lips. I see that same sparkle when I am teasing you. We share the same thoughts with unspoken words.

I found in her someone that accepted me. She loved me as myself—not wanting to change me in any way...except no butter on the green beans of course.

I found myself smitten.

She never had to open a door in my presence again. This surprised Maureen. I surprised myself. She just had such a humble demeanor that made you want to treat her better than she treated herself. Opening the door for her (every time for the rest of our lives together) simply felt right. This smallest of gestures just cemented what we meant to each other.

More comically, I made her a mixed tape of love songs since nobody had told me in 1997 that those went out in the eighties. She liked it anyway. I spliced together a video of forty big-screen kisses, but I later realized that *Gone with the Wind* and *Die Hard* did not belong on the same video. For her birthday, I took winter photos of our favorite Portland haunts and made her stationery and a journal with those photos.

> *Lovers know that snowflakes melt with*
> *changes in the weather, but*
> *Memories made in the snow*
> *will stay with them forever.*

Maureen had started a collection of materials to make cards for everyone in her life as part of healing those relationships. She experimented with mixed media and had bags and bags of dried flowers and lace and ribbons and varieties of papers. She used ink stamps. She tried coloring with pencils and pastels and oil sticks. She sent some my way, and they remain treasures still.

I would email her at work and vice versa. We would use pseudonyms at first so those in Eugene did not know who she wrote. I often addressed them to my Pretty Lady and signed from her Dearheart. She had never much liked her name "Maureen" and said she got teased in school, or people would not hear it right and think it was Marie and then always tell her, "You don't look like a Marie." For a while I made up the name Annie. It made her giggle. It stuck for years. She started to transcend the pain of her yesterdays.

As I rise above the strife,
I understand one more dimension
Of love and life.

By offering daily
Caring, listening, laughter, tears
By sharing unfailingly

All which mirrors hope.
Hope, the recipe of life
The rest of your years

A reassuring touch, a warm smile,
A gentle kiss.
I will love you forever, eternally.
            Maureen Patrick, April 1997

Maureen introduced me to church after nearly thirty years of casual acquaintance with the institution (I had gone to Sunday School as a kid to support a teacher-friend of my mother's). When in Eugene, Maureen and I went to the Faith Center every Sunday. She preferred this Christian Foursquare Church. They practiced a practical application of God's lessons in your everyday life. They practiced forgiveness and not judgment. That pleased her, as Maureen judged herself plenty.

On June 1, 1997, she and I had spent the weekend at her apartment in Eugene and went to the church that morning. They announced a baptism for that evening. Later that day, Maureen turned to me and said, "I want to get baptized tonight. I think that is important at this point in my life. I was baptized when I was younger, but I've made a lot of bad decisions since then, and I want to start my life anew."

"Can I assume that I am a part of that new life?" I asked.

"Yes, you are. I asked God to either put you in my life or take you out of it, and he put you into it."

We remained quiet for a bit, listening to some music and sitting together drinking tea in her living room.

"Would you like me to get baptized too?" I asked her.

"It has to be your decision. You have to do it for you," she replied.

"Well, you've introduced me to church these last five months. It feels right to me, and I want to make a commitment. If you do not mind, I want to do this together." She hugged and kissed me, and I knew that she wanted that too.

That night, we arrived at the church and Pastor Steve explained what would happen. Eight of us were to be baptized. I stood in a dressing room with an older man and a young boy not more than seven years old. Maureen had four women with her. We changed into white garments with our clothes on underneath and dry ones set aside for after. As we assembled behind the stage, Maureen wanted me to come up to stand right behind her, so I did.

Pastor Steve took me aside and said, "Scott I am glad you are doing this. There is a lady who is on the large side being baptized tonight. She wants to be lowered three times. For her safety, I am wondering if I can place her right after you, so after you are baptized, could you stay in the water and help me with her? I don't want to be struggling, and I want her to feel comfortable."

I said, "Of course." Maureen overheard and smiled with a tear in her eye. This told her heart that we had made the right choices.

We came out on stage. Two people received their baptism before Maureen, then she walked up. She welcomed it, calm and reserved, but elated. She looked at me and smiled before she went under and again when she came out, even more so.

My turn came, and I found a joy and peace and contentment in it all. I had never been baptized and now I followed a woman who, in just a few months of being together, had become the love of my life. I descended, then rose. I remained, and together Pastor Steve and I lowered and raised the woman who stood after me three times. We got out of the water together, and I stood with Maureen. We took a step together, blessing our relationship.

Our love continued to grow. I would write her notes and stick them in her overnight bag. I started a journal and would write a few pages, then hand it to her for her to write a few more pages and hand it back. We filled it with our thoughts and love and prayers for each other.

Shared Journal: Scott to Maureen – July 28, 1997

We have found in each other the best we will ever find. You and I will never know greater love. Hold onto that thought, and you will be set free of your fears. When I say I love, adore, cherish, and will spend the rest of my life spoiling you and that I will enjoy every minute of it, I mean it. I mean it forever because that is just how I'm made."

Shared Journal: Maureen to Scott – July 30, 1997

I am in love with you, and yes, there are lingering fears from my past. I know you love me and always will. If our love were not true, we would not have survived these seven months, nor come together after the year apart during my darkest times. I want this opportunity that God has given me. He found, and put, a person in my life who is like me. I have never found anyone else to understand my sense of humor, much less the giggles I get. I have never had anyone

We shared these kinds of heartfelt words back and forth in writing, over the phone, or in person. Sometimes she deviated from the romantic. She would also continue to impart words of wisdom to me. She had reading glasses and cleaned them by using the hem of her sweater. Once, I reached for a tissue and offered it up. She comically provided the life lesson, "Never use a tissue on glass. That will scratch it. You might as well use a log." To this day, I typically carry a cloth handkerchief in my pocket and think about that comment.

Maureen had decided she would move up to Portland after the end of the year. She loved her children and grandchild immensely, but the job had proved a drudgery. I offered to leave my job and move down, but she wanted to be up in Portland with more to see and do. She knew we would travel down often to see the kids, but they became increasingly busier with their own lives. She craved change. She also thought we should save money and someday get a house together. While we had expressed our love many times, we had not discussed marriage as yet, nor did it seem a topic she ever gravitated toward. She wanted to remain together for always yes, but also had an attitude of, "let us not ruin it." I did not mention it.

She thought an ideal way to save money included just renting a room from her friend Jeanne in Portland. I had only met her and her husband a couple of times—nice people sure enough, but I had some trepidation of moving into a room in their home. Maureen had spoken to Jeanne, and they had known each other for over forty years. They would do anything for each other.

We planned for my move in November, and Maureen would come in January. I would live in a single bedroom of her friend's house without Maureen for two months. "Awkward" came to mind. They had a wonderful attitude and made me feel at ease. Still, I spent a lot of time out of the home to give them their privacy and slowly transition into it. Maureen came two months later, and we stayed in a single bedroom with our things in a small storage unit a couple of miles away. The bedroom came furnished, so we stored almost everything. The room included a waterbed. Neither of us had ever slept in a waterbed. Jeanne's husband assured us that it would do wonders for our backs. Maureen and I giggled so hard that first night sloshing around.

We lived there for fourteen months. They remain great friends, but that felt like a loooooong fourteen months in one bedroom: yes, in a waterbed.

We worked full time and loved to take walks, grab a bite on the waterfront, or take in some live music. As such, it gave our friends time alone too in their home. We would eat with them a couple of nights a week or go out for Dim Sum and help them with some odd jobs around the house. Really, though, we tried to keep our footprint there small. We shared the bathroom with Jeanne's teenage son, who seemed to take it all in his stride and spent most of his time on video games in his room. We did eventually advocate for a single kitchen cupboard for when we ate in.

Maureen had gotten a job with the city transportation company, Tri-Met, as a bus driver. She did the training and then got cold feet. Portland proved a lot bigger than Eugene. With so many unfamiliar areas to learn, the task seemed too daunting. She had known Eugene like the back of her hand. She told me she wanted to quit and got a job in an office for an insurance company.

When my work schedule allowed, we would take the light rail into work together. I would walk her to the door of her building holding hands and leave her with a very public kiss and hug. Often after work, we would linger downtown with walks along the waterfront or catching dinner somewhere new. We saw art and listened to music and window shopped. She finally had some of the experiences that she craved.

We celebrated this chapter in both of our lives, but still faced hurdles. Her daughter, even after our year together, still did not accept me. The way Maureen had left her first husband (their father) cut deeply. Her daughter had never reconciled for herself why Maureen had done what she did—the way she had. Despite numerous apologies and explanations by Maureen, her daughter could not yet fully forgive or trust. She wanted to shelter herself and her family from that kind of hurt again. Would I simply be gone one day too and leave them with more emotional shrapnel in my wake?

That first Christmas required patience. The family time and celebrations had to happen on their terms to build that trust back. I desperately wanted to spend that first Christmas with Maureen but was not allowed in her daughter's house. Instead, I stayed at a nearby hotel and had Christmas Eve dinner alone at a late-night buffet.

Maureen felt guilty leaving me to go to her daughter's home, but we also agreed on the necessity of these smaller steps. She enjoyed the festivities with her daughter (now pregnant a second time), her son-in-law, and that darling first grandchild. She returned to me late that night in the hotel, where I had set up a small eighteen-inch artificial tree with a burlap base, bow, a single strand of lights, and a few mini ornaments. I also had three gifts for her under that tree. Maureen could not stop smiling at the surprise. We set up that tree in our bedroom every year thereafter.

Her son had accepted us far more readily. He had a "live and let live" nature about him. He and Maureen had healed much of their relationship. He simply wanted his mother happy.

We navigated the cold reception from her daughter's family best we could. Maureen (or often both of us) would still regularly go down to Eugene to see her kids and grandkids, as the second one had arrived by then. She now had a beautiful granddaughter too.

Shared Journal: from Maureen – 4/1/98

No foolin'. It was so nice to come home. I had not realized how much Jeanne's house really is home, at least for the time being. I attribute most of it to you. You made everything so special: the flowers, cards, coffee, clean sheets, and all the little touches I care so much about. I love being with my daughter and her growing family, but it is evident it is her home. I clearly am a visitor, which is ok. I enjoyed my time, but I was ready to return here.

I missed you. Have I told you today how much I love you? It should be an everyday occurrence. Thanks for all you do and all you are in my life.

I love the lyrics you wrote, and when things settle down a bit, I will write in the notes or at least the melody. I do not believe I am qualified to write a full score.

You are an incredible person, and yes, we are so much alike from the little things to the big things to the Dairy Queen Blizzards. I promise to clean up the clutter from my "projects".

After being at both my son's and daughter's, I am really glad to see that they are with partners who have common interests. I bet my approach to things drove them crazy. You understand. You and I share my silly sense of humor.

Thank you for being you and being a part of my life.

All my love kept right in my heart.

Annie

While our personal life included much of what we wanted, Maureen's office job only lasted three months. It made her miserable. Perhaps it was too much like the old office job. After all those years, she still enjoyed driving bus. She liked being outside but not IN the weather. Maureen liked her interaction with so many diverse and interesting people. She wanted to go back and give the bus driving another chance. I sent her flowers on her last day at the office, and that made her, and all the other ladies, smile. Again, everyone liked her wherever she went—she just lacked confidence.

She retrained with Tri-Met and became a driver. Earlier, she wanted to change her name: new town, new start. She first trained as Renee. She even had her name legally changed. She had never liked her real name: the mispronunciation, misspelling, and teasing she endured as a kid had shaken her confidence. However, after a few weeks she realized that a name change would solve nothing. She held old baggage from her childhood. As such, she legally changed her name back to Maureen before the second training. I supported her decision-making and did not offer counsel. I tried to respect her choices rather than shoot her down.

As such, some drivers knew her as Renee and others as Maureen.

Bus driving at Tri-Met means you bid routes every quarter. You get assigned a sign-up time, and you pick your first, second, and third preferred routes based on what remains on the board. Maureen wanted to stay in the SE side where she had learned her way around and tried to get one of the weekend days off to maximize our time together. I would advise her on the sketchier parts of town to avoid. Each quarter, I would drive the route with her to get her familiar with it before she had to do it for real in the bus. The first few times, she had to pull a Saturday evening, so I would ride with her to keep her company and bring her dinner. We made it work—we made them memorable times.

Life

To be joyous, not bitter.
To be shared, not lonely.
To be reveled, not wasted.
To do and live is
To nurture your soul.

Sew your dreams,
And wear them
Like a winter coat
That keeps you warm
And lets you brave the cold world.

Seek out comfort in it all,
And find that which
Makes you smile,
Warms your heart,
And provides you love and caring.

Hold these things close,
And let them fill your senses,
For they make life worth living.
That kind of living is truly
What life is about.

Scott to Maureen

Confidence proved difficult for Maureen to find throughout most of her life. She had been plagued with anxiety attacks for years over prior and current choices. She judged herself harder than anyone around her. Daily, we would talk about what she had accomplished that day, no matter how big or small. Together we tried to build a collection of accomplishments to shield that fragile ego.

Despite these struggles, she did slowly gain confidence in her driving. She drove defensively and had a mind for the details. She had done it for years in Eugene, and now here. She ventured to signing other runs, including the summer Washington Park route. She shuttled people between the Oregon Zoo, Arboretum, Japanese Garden, and Rose Gardens (all favorites of ours). She perhaps enjoyed that run most with the people that would ride it from all over the world. This did not typically include the people with the morning or afternoon drudgery of work, rather people vacationing and taking in the Portland sites. She thrived in that environment, despite her otherwise shy demeanor. They treated her like a tour guide, and that gave her a confidence boost.

In April of 1999, we bought our own home in SE Portland and moved out of Jeanne's house. The new house (an English Tudor from the late 1940s) appealed to our simple nature, but with a little style. We could move in as is, but it certainly needed some work. The prior owner had taken a wallpapering class and used her home to test her skills…many times…many, many times. They had some…failed applications.

Neither Maureen nor I had ever remodeled a home, but we felt sure we could figure it out together. First, we stripped the wallpaper. In some cases, they had applied as many as seven layers. We then would prep and paint the walls, then replace the flooring. As it turned out, after stripping the wallpaper, we found we had to patch the plaster walls. The prior owner had damaged many of the walls, and she had filled the holes with newspaper and covered them with cardboard before wallpapering. Apparently, she had not taken the plastering class too.

We replaced appliances, ran gas and electrical, replaced light fixtures, tried our hands at tiling, and far more. We had many a mishap, but never one argument. We loved discovering this process together, and she felt confident in that I learned right along with her.

We laughed and enjoyed it and made it our home. I made sure we broke the work up with outings to concerts, galleries, long walks on the waterfront, farmer's markets, and weekend getaways. Sometimes the planner part of me went into overdrive. I remember one weekend specifically when I came up with four or five different things we could do. As I presented them, she turned each one down. Finally, a little flustered, I asked, "Well then what DO you want to do?" She smiled calmly and said, "Just spend time with you." She did that for me. She helped me slow down. She helped me realize not everything needed a plan.

We got a cat together. We bought a lot of holiday decorations for each of the seasons. For the first several months, we lived as a married couple, although we were not. That worried Maureen from two perspectives: she felt we should marry if we lived together but at the same time was deathly afraid of getting married again.

December 1999, after being in the house for about eight months, Maureen's demeanor changed. We had lived as a couple for three years and known each other six and a half at this point. She had sudden reservations about us sleeping together after three years of doing so. She asked that I move to the adjacent bedroom. I asked if I had done something, but she said no. I asked why, but she refused to talk about it. She said she had reservations about "it all" but would give no further details.

Not having developed that depth of understanding yet, I sulked but did as she asked. We still held hands and did things together, but a wedge now sat between us. I did not understand. I tried not to push her, as I did not want to shake the confidence she had developed, but this seemed neither fair nor right. Her old fears of two failed marriages had returned.

She had often driven down to see her kids on her days off to remain close to them. This increased after the purchase of the house. I missed our fun times. Outings I had planned our first year together now got cancelled more times than not for something with the kids. I missed the earlier "just spend time with you" sentiment. I told myself that maybe I loved more deeply than she did.

To make things worse, I did the thing that had now become cliché in relationships. I especially should have known better. I spoke to a woman at work about my concerns with the struggles in my relationship with Maureen. This lady had struggles of her own in hers. She described it as an "ongoing divorce" in which they frequently went through the separation process but stalled at the final stage. I told myself, "This woman listens to me. She gets me. She supports me." I made bad choices—textbook.

I still tried with Maureen. I tried to reason why we had this sudden wedge between us and thought, even though she did not speak of it, maybe she wanted to get married. Valentine's Day approached. I thought maybe a proposal would change things. To this day, I do not know if Maureen could tell what I had planned or simply went to the next stage of her shaken confidence. A week before Valentine's Day 2000, she told me in an abrupt manner, not even sitting me down to talk, "Don't ever ask me to marry you because I don't want to have to tell you no."

I had never loved someone nearly as much as Maureen (nor have I since). She remains the only person who I ever considered marrying. However, I was upset that she had just tore my heart apart in such a dismissive way. We had loved each other in our actions and words. We had shared countless beautiful notes and sentiments. I did not have the experience or maturity to see the pain and fear she still carried. She would not talk about it either. I started to give up.

I lamented on everything for a month and started to distance myself. I told all this to the other woman—a good woman. I should not have done that. In one ear, Maureen told me that we had no future, and in the other, another woman told me all the things I wanted to hear. I would never describe this good woman as manipulative. She was just hurting too from her own on-again, off-again marriage.

I made a rash and regrettable decision, and I left Maureen. We both cried harder than we had ever cried, and we each cried alone. I put up hard walls, so she could not talk me out of it. I made a series of bad choices.

I moved out and left Maureen the house and most of our things. I agreed to keep paying half of everything 'till we figured out what we wanted to do. This occurred just a few weeks before her fiftieth birthday. She was alone again. We had not married, but this hurt her no less than her divorces. In fact, it hurt far more so because unlike the other two times, she knew she still loved me. She just did not know how to explain what she felt, and I did not understand to stick it out.

I did an odd thing. While I apologized to Maureen, I did the same with all her family. I wrote her kids, her mother, her friends, and other family. Anybody in her life that I met, I wrote them and apologized. I told them Maureen had done nothing wrong—that I did this. I apologized repeatedly and asked them to not leave her alone, but to look after her. I just tried patching my own guilt.

For three months, I stayed away, save for the monthly check and continued apologies in brief notes to Maureen. I spent that time with the other woman (now divorced): again, a good person but troubled as well. Every part of my old life I just pushed away. I frantically tried to make a new one. Those I worked with started to talk—unsure what to think of my personality shift. I started thinking only about me and what I wanted. I did not understand at the time that I had created a large hole in my life and was trying to fill that void. I did not understand that I would never fill it with all that I grabbed for. I still made my own bad choices.

Maureen started out sad and isolating but then replayed everything that had happened and became determined.

Maureen's Journal – 4/4/00

I can see that I was too preoccupied with the past than the present, and I realize I was not paying enough attention to the person that I love most and not intertwining him with my family. I talk so much of just healing my own family. That healing has started, but at what cost?...

I need to write a book from all the beautiful cards and letters and journals. I cannot imagine anyone else having so many beautiful passages. I was one of the most blessed people on the face of the world. Has anyone been loved so much? Or loved so much? . . .

> We were meant for always. This is not about me. He helped me along, but I truly believe we both want the same thing. I want a marriage of commitment. Scott and I could have had that, and we still can, even more so now...
>
> He is my one true love and I love him with my heart and soul. He is all that matters. Now is the time for me to respect his wishes and pray that God works in his life. My poor soul mate is hurting desperately. For two years, he has been on the back burner and expected to understand.
>
> I will call Rosemary to set up an appointment to process the other issues besides guilt and shame. I have to conquer fear, not through control, but through trust and love. I have to relax my mind. Scott always loved me for who I was. He is hurting now...

She had a beautiful, forgiving, graceful, and understanding soul, but blamed herself too much.

With me absent, she spent more time with family to seek comfort. She lunched with her hundred-and-two-year-old great aunt Rose and travelled down to see her kids and grandbabies. She had talks with her mother trying to figure out what went wrong. She cried with her good friends—her lifelong girlfriends—to come to terms with what had happened. But none of it felt enough. She did not want to give up on us.

In June on my birthday, Maureen left a gift on the doorstep of my apartment. She included a card:

Dearheart –

Your own true beliefs come from the heart...
Be true to your heart.
Beliefs of others,
About whom you should be
Cause doubt, and are just from the mind...
I pray for strength of
Character for you
So that you may emerge your true
Self to honor the Lord.
May you have many blessings
On your 33rd birthday.

Annie & Maureen
I am the same

She also included a gift card for a video rental. She wrote on the sleeve, "For *Jerry Maguire*": our first date.

The new girlfriend found the gift first. It made her distraught. She saw Maureen trying to repair things to get me back. I unconvincingly tried to ease her fears. She knew I still loved Maureen.

I went to church alone a couple of nights later. They had no service that night, but they let me in. The hall sat empty save for a few people doing business. This Foursquare Church Maureen and I used to go to east of Portland now felt like my only safe haven, though I entered with shame. We had gone to church regularly. We really enjoyed this particular church family with Pastor Ted and the good people we had met along the way. I had gone to two men's retreats to develop that relationship with God. We had done so much spiritual soul-searching and committed to each other. Now, I saw it all unravel before me—all my own doing.

Alone, I asked God to either put Maureen in my life or take her out of it, just as Maureen had done almost four years prior. God did not give me the same kind of answer he gave Maureen. Maureen still remained in my life. I needed to make the decision, and He refused to make it easy on me.

I left the other woman. We had tears, and she was angry too. She threw things at me. I deserved her anger. I had never broken off a relationship in my life, and I had just done it with two people within four months of each other. I had strayed so far from the path that I needed to follow.

Broken and with complete humility, I asked Maureen to meet me for dinner. This kind and gracious woman accepted my request. We started dinner at 4 p.m. that Saturday. I did not get her home 'till after midnight. We talked about everything. I apologized again. I told her every detail of why I left. I told her about the other woman. I told her I never stopped loving her but had seen no future for us. I said that it seemed like nothing that I had done in those years could break through. I then shut up and listened.

Maureen went way back. She told me of her abuse as a child by her grandfather. She told me in far more detail than she had before about the pain and humiliation in her first and second marriages. She had hinted at these things before but always cut herself off before going deeper. Things that she had not told anyone, or very few people, she told me now and made herself completely vulnerable.

She told me she loved me too much to let those mistakes of her past happen with us anymore. She then told me that during our time apart she had come to understand that she was still living with old fears. She understood that we would not fail in our marriage because we started from a better place. We used this dinner as one small part of that better place. We had a good evening.

"She is a beautiful piece of broken pottery, put back together by her own hands. And a critical world judges her cracks while missing the beauty of how she made herself whole again." — J.M. Storm

I did not understand that before. I understood now.

When I dropped her off, we remained quiet but giggled. Her mother and stepfather slept in the daylit basement of the house. They had helped her fix it up while I had made all my stupid, bad decisions. They lived in a motor home year-round, but they remained up here in the summer before snow-birding down south. They stayed there to keep her company.

I dropped off this beautiful, fifty-year-old woman at her home after midnight with her mother in the house. Oddly, a house I still half-owned. Maureen and I kissed. I laughed at the odd position I now found myself in and drove away. About a mile out, I turned around and went back, now close to one in the morning. I found some pebbles on the street and went to the side of the house and threw them at her bedroom window. I saw her light on, as she had not yet gone to sleep. She went to the window and looked down at me.

"What are you doing you goof?"

"I love you. I've never stopped loving you," I shout-whispered.

She giggled. "I love you too."

I stared back up at this most beautiful woman. "I'll love you always—always and one day more."

She smiled, "Always and one day more."

I knew we healed a lot that night. We had a good evening.

Four months later we married. We found more happiness than we had ever known.

Chapter 4

Marriage

M arriage, they say, requires a lot of work. I have never enjoyed a job more.

While we dated (and reinforced after our reunion), Maureen explained what she wanted in a relationship. We walked along the waterfront that summer and talked about it.

She started, "I spent too much of my first two marriages as a low priority. We will both have jobs, and yours requires some travel and some evenings. I do not want you to give that up. But when you are not working, I want you to make me the priority. When your work is done, I want you to rush home to me because you want to be with me. If you ask to go have drinks with friends or co-workers, then I am not the priority. Work is work—I get it. But we have no kids at home, very few friends, and we have gone through a lot to be together. I have to know I will be the priority."

I listened. I sensed she had more to say so did not interrupt.

She continued, "You know I am not good with strangers or at parties or stuff like that. I think I will get better, but, for now, it is hard for me. When we have to go to those, I want you by my side. I do not want to be left alone in a corner. I cannot stop being a priority for you in those situations. I need to matter to you—always."

Maureen took and cradled my arm. I could see that she said this lovingly, not accusatory. She said I had already shown her that kind of attention over the prior three plus years. She said it like a speech she felt she should have given before her first marriage or her second. She did not want this relationship to have any misunderstandings.

I could see the commitment in her eyes and hear it in her voice. I saw that she had replaced her earlier fears of marriage with trust.

I promised her.

I had never bought a ring before. I went to a jeweler on a recommendation from a friend. You pick the ring first, then you pick the center diamond, and they join the two. I recalled that my mother had a two-piece ring. The engagement one had the center stone and then another one fit together with it. I knew Maureen loved traditional gold and diamonds. She preferred traditional, understated elegance and quality over flash or "getting noticed". All her life, she preferred simplicity and modesty.

I figured she deserved more than just a single diamond. I opted for a large center diamond with a few little diamonds around it— after all, her April birthday meant a diamond birthstone. Funds caused me to settle on a half carat center stone, traditional cut, but I opted for a higher quality. I figured in the future I could change to a larger stone. We did just that on our ten-year anniversary when we renewed our vows and upgraded to a full carat.

On September 1, 2000, I took Maureen to a favorite park of ours up in the west hills with the ring hidden in my pocket. I had not revealed the purpose of our trip. We sat on a bench late afternoon with very few people in the area. I had prepared what I wanted to say and knelt down on one knee.

"I love you. Yes, I really love you.
I love you to the core of my being.
I know it in my soul. I know it in my heart.
I think about you, and I think about us all the time.
I truly know that I want to spend the rest of my life with you.

In Song of Solomon, *the man tells his bride to be,*
"You are all fair, my love, and there is no spot in you."
He is saying that he sees her as pure.
The love in his heart has made her the perfect bride for him.
That is how I see you.

I want to be everything to you that I can.
I want to be everything that you never had and everything
you always wanted.
I want to love you the rest of my days.
I want to still be your best friend and your Dearheart,
But I also want to be your husband.

Will you marry me?"

Happily, she said yes, and we celebrated at a favorite restaurant of ours. She could not stop looking at the ring. I brought the other half too, so she could see it together. She loved it and commented many times to me, and friends, that she could not believe how perfectly the ring fit her personality.

We planned the wedding ourselves and got it done in three months. She wanted a smaller wedding but still traditional. She wanted the wedding to take place in the winter: hence the short engagement. She asked her longtime friend Candy to stand as her matron of honor and another dear friend, Mary, to make her wedding dress. Maureen asked her to include white velour for the bodice and satin for the rest. Her conservative nature commanded sleeves, a high neck, and simple lines. She looked stunning. Flowers in the winter consisted of evergreen boughs and Calla Lilies, except for her bouquet, which included white roses with pink edges. Those colors represented the sentiment "I will love you always." My boutonniere matched.

We picked a small church from the mid 1800s. A group had wanted to preserve it from developers and floated it down the river to its current site. This saved the charming building. Nothing could have looked more like a traditional church. It sat modestly, all white with a steeple and stained glass.

The pews held only about sixty people total, so we kept the invite list short. To stem the ire of the extended family that we did not invite to the ceremony, we invited them to the reception afterwards two blocks away. Still, as few believed Maureen would marry again or that I would ever marry, the weather cooperated, and many stood in the front yard with the doors propped open. They peered in throughout the ceremony. Afterward, the entire party made their way to the reception hall.

We took care of almost everything ourselves with a little help on the final touches the day before from our closest family and friends. With Maureen at fifty and me at thirty-three, we understood the arrangements rested with us. This helped it to align with our style.

Yes, we danced.

Yes, Maureen remained completely happy and content throughout the day. She knew almost everyone there well and could feel at ease with them. Her kids attended, and by then her daughter had three children. Maureen's first grandson, now at four and a half, enjoyed bearing the ring. Her first granddaughter, at two and a half, agreed to fill the role of flower girl, and their recently new baby brother, at just three weeks old, did what babies do. Even with the familiarity of friends and family, I stayed at Maureen's side throughout, making sure she remained at ease.

We provided dinner for all. We had cake…politely with no face smushing. I would look at my wife throughout the afternoon and early evening and thought how beautiful and happy she looked. I felt blessed.

The guests cleared out and we cleaned up a bit faster than I had assumed we would. I stalled a bit, raising some suspicion. As we loaded the last of the stuff, a Rolls Royce that I had arranged pulled up to take Maureen and I on a drive around the city for the evening lights. Maureen relished this surprise. She felt elegant, classy, and very loved. We danced in the park where I proposed.

We honeymooned in San Francisco for a week, which became a travel favorite of ours. On that trip, we committed to returning every five years on our anniversary, and we did.

I understood that I had such an amazing wife. She loved spending time with me. She encouraged me to plan adventures. She stayed flexible when things did not go right and could laugh about it. She had a limitless ability to love family and friends. She stayed true to herself and lovingly accepted me "as is". Her quiet, reserved, and simple nature showed off her elegance, thoughtfulness, and growing comfort in her own skin. She did not crave the center of attention but certainly sat squarely in the center of my world. I told her numerous times each day that I loved her. She said that warmed her heart, but not as much as when I told her, "I'll be home on time tonight." To have someone want to spend so much time with you feels pretty wonderful.

HITYTHMILY?

Have I told you today how much I love you?

We always put that in our cards and notes to each other.

As noted earlier, our home that we bought in early Spring 1999 had a 1940s English Tudor style. It seemed as though we never stopped remodeling. We kept exploring things together. We kept it new and exciting.

We ended up adding floorboards for storage in the rafters. We added a laundry chute that the grandkids loved to test. They would take wash cloths and drop them down the chute, run to the laundry basket in the basement to retrieve them, and run back up to do it again. Apparently, hours of fun. We also had a mail slot in the side of the house. The postman dropped mail through it into a basket in the coat closet off the foyer. We handed the grandkids envelopes for the novelty of it. This also provided great entertainment.

We got cats. We got a lot of cats. Prior to marriage, we got one long-haired Himalayan, Mandy, that comforted Maureen during our four months apart. Sadly, shortly after we got back together and before getting married, a neighbor's dog got loose and severed poor Mandy's arm. That required us to put her down.

Maureen took a while to get over that loss but then offered to get me a cat for my birthday. I knew the real intent. She had turned a corner and found herself ready to have another cat.

We went back to the humane society and found a similar long-haired breed, though a darker, smokey gray, and we named her Misty. Misty started out friendly but liked her independence. At the first opportunity, she bolted. We struggled to find her and bring her back. We would set food outside with the hope of enticing her. Someone ate it—Misty or strays. With a dutiful eye, we kept watch for her, but we rarely caught a glimpse. However, one summer evening as we were lying in bed, I looked out the window and saw Misty on the neighbor's roof staring back at me. The next morning, Misty had vanished, but she left a…"present" on our neighbor's roof.

Bad kitty. We never told the neighbors, and the next rain took care of it. Well, I imagine until they cleaned the gutters.

Not wanting to both have a cat and not REALLY have a cat, Maureen took in two kittens from her son, whose cat had a litter. She grabbed two simple gray tabbies whom she promptly named Buddy and Missy My. She informed me all cats named by her had Ys at the end of their names. This made it easier to call them. Once these kittens got a bit older, we let them out too. We had pet doors in the detached garage and at the back-kitchen door. With training, they ran in and out all the time. Misty apparently noticed the new residents and all of a sudden started coming around more and even back into the house. As such, we now had three cats.

Two years later, while reading the morning paper, Maureen made the comment that she had always liked calico cats: specifically, their coloring. She had fond memories of the calico cat she had when she was a girl, Tiger. I said nothing and read my section of the paper. Clueless, I did not pick up that she had more to share. She then elaborated by saying that she had seen an ad for two available calico mixes in the paper.

I asked if we could get just one, and she agreed. However, getting there, the person let us know they had to go as a pair. "Of course," I thought. So we had two more new kittens to train. One of them proved quite the explorer. She nearly fell into a juniper bush by jumping out of my hands before we could even get them in the car. I reactively caught her by the tail just in time and got a firmer hold. I noticed her tail had a bend and was worried that I had just done that. The owner assured me that kitten had caught its tail in a door two days prior. That one got the name Lucky and her sister Lady for the comparatively dainty way she carried herself. Yes, we now had five cats. This made Maureen very happy.

A couple of years later on a Saturday morning, we thought we heard a noise in the garage. We had just started the paper and coffee when the noise startled us both. "Can you go see what that is?" Maureen asked.

In slippers, underwear, and a robe, I ventured out and up the drive to the garage. I opened the door and switched on the light. I started counting cats. All five had climbed up on worktops and counters. I followed Buddy's eyes to the food dish and saw a large opossum eating their food. I thought, "Great". I shut off the light, closed the door, went back inside, and sat down to drink my coffee and read the paper.

"What was the noise?" Maureen asked. "Are they all ok?"

"Yeah. It's just an opossum." I sipped my coffee.

She paused. "Well, where is it?"

"I left it in the garage," I dismissed. "It'll eat a little and be on its way."

"No, it won't!" Maureen had knowledge of such critters. She had battled opossums and raccoons out in the country in her younger life. I always learned something new about her. "It will keep coming back as long as there's food. It will attack the cats if it gets threatened. You have to kill it."

I put down my coffee and looked at my calm, kind, and gentle wife—the woman who loved all animals telling me that I now needed to kill one. She continued, "You don't understand honey. It will bring friends. We'll get overrun, and the cats will have to come indoors."

"Well then, you go ahead and kill it," I said. I thought that would end my involvement. Such a silly man.

Feeling a stare at my temple, I turned to meet my wife's eyes. I did not know that eyes could smirk. "What?! I have to kill it?!" I asked.

"Yes," she giggled. Maureen would not do it even though she had killed all sorts of birds and varmints as a kid in central Oregon. She had fired many a shotgun at chukars, gophers, and more. I had never killed anything but an ant pile as a kid. I admit I felt squeamish.

Thinking better than starting an argument against it, I went back out. The cats were still on their counters and kept staring at the unwanted guest who continued nibbling their food. I put on the light, and the opossum froze and looked at me with one beady eye. I had no idea what to do. I stood there in my underwear, robe, and slippers and looked around the garage for something to kill the opossum with.

I saw a shovel hanging on the wall. I removed it, and the cats all scurried out of the garage. Apparently, they either worried that I had come for them or figured out what I had planned to do and did not want to bear witness. Completely lost on process and still squeamish, I reasoned that I could just smack it on the head really hard and kill it that way.

The opossum had not yet moved, still watching me with one eye. I positioned myself next to it and reached out with the shovel, hovering it over the beast's head. I raised it up, turned and squinted, and smacked it down as hard as I could. Cat food went flying, and the opossum lay under the shovel head. I lifted the end, and the opossum showed its teeth and growled at me.

Oh no, oh no. Panic now started in. I swung the shovel again and only got a glancing blow as the opossum took off, running through the garage, out the door, and into the vegetable garden. Maureen had planted marigolds all around the perimeter to keep the slugs away. Overgrown and in full bloom, the marigolds proved a good hiding spot, and the opossum ducked in there. It stayed very still. I circled above it on the slightly raised deck and peered over the railing. With the end of the shovel, I parted each cluster of marigolds 'till I saw fur. I thought, "Ok, with this angle, I will need to rest the point of the shovel on the back of its neck and then just push down."

As I positioned it, a shred of reason took hold for only a moment, "Let's make sure this isn't one of the cats."

I confirmed—opossum. It remained very still, hoping I would go away, or perhaps even still stunned from the earlier smackdown. I repositioned the shovel blade, turned and squinted again, and drove it down. I looked down and saw that the head of the opossum was now turned 180 degrees, like Regan MacNeil. It looked up the shovel handle at me and growled again. With continued panic, I raised and drove the shovel down again and again a few times 'till I knew I had completed my grisly task.

I left the shovel there in the garden and went inside. I washed my hands, poured a fresh cup of coffee, and sat down in the front room to restart the paper. Maureen had not moved but watched my actions. Still looking at the paper, I said, "It's done".

After a long pause with Maureen's inquisitive stare very much piercing my temple, she asked, "Where is it?"

"I did as you asked and killed it. It's dead in the vegetable garden."

"Well you have to get rid of it," she explained.

"Yes, later. After my coffee and paper and getting dressed," I countered. I read on a minute or two but felt that familiar stare.

I looked over. "Now?"

"Yes please," she giggled again.

"I love you," I confirmed with a look and a smirk.

"I know," she grinned.

Insisting on putting on pants first, I then ventured back out and disposed of the beast.

This lays out our marriage well—not the opossum killing, (though I became known for years by others in the family as the great hunter), but the yin and yang of direction and action. She had a vision, and I executed the plan (perhaps poor words in respect to the opossum). I remained hopelessly in love with my wife and really had not become so set in my ways as to argue. She loved that she finally had a voice in a relationship. She loved that her opinion mattered.

All forms of things in our marriage had that sort of relationship: loving and supportive, but direction and action.

She had a vision for the house remodeling and the colors. She asked my opinion, but in the end, I always let her decide. With dinner, banking, vacations, decorations, or whatever, we approached it all the same.

She loved the holidays and, in her words, "finally got to decorate big." I admittedly fell easily into that role, especially at Christmas when we went all out.

Her wanting to go big meant lots of lights. She loved Christmas lights. She also wanted decorations on the walls and trees. She placed some sort of precious heirloom piece on what seemed like every horizontal surface in the house.

I took "big" to translate into the physical size as well. She helped with the exterior but left most of that to me. Over the years, the decorations became more elaborate, with a handmade train in the front yard filled with stuffed animals. We had a nativity scene that eventually had to get a substitute baby Jesus. That year in Portland, many yards experienced a rash of Jesus thefts.

We had a small, covered porch out front that I would turn into a Santa's workshop. Given the prior theft and the gorge wind, I attached plexiglas to the front and sides so people could see in, but not remove items. I included an animated Santa, toys, and elves. The plexiglas also kept the childlike elves from blowing into the driveway (not a good look). I then split the scene with the addition of an animated snowman singing with a reindeer and a penguin.

This first home of ours sat across the street from a Catholic senior care facility. Each year, the weekend after Thanksgiving, a handful of seniors would set up folding chairs in their front yard and watch me work away setting up the decorations. I would get unsolicited pointers but always taken with joy and levity.

On the interior, Maureen really shined.

Her fondest Christmas memories as a child included her father taking a vacuum to flock the tree. Back in the day, you could switch your vacuum to run in reverse. He would put flocking in the vacuum and self-flock a tree. It created a beautiful tree that looked covered in snow, but it also ruined more than one of their vacuums.

For that reason, I thought better to buy a pre-flocked tree than create one. For those who have never bought a real flocked tree, your finances likely remain intact. After a couple of years of over-priced tree lots, we explored other options. Boring, Oregon (yes you read that right) is a small, remote, rural town that includes Dutcher's Farm.

There, you can cut your own green tree, but they also have a couple dozen pre-flocked trees in the barn. These amazingly kind people also keep their flocked trees very reasonably priced. Given the bargain, Maureen felt compelled each year to also get a couple of flocked wreaths, a flocked centerpiece for the dining room table, and a bird feeder the older gentlemen made. A good friend once asked me if I ever told Maureen no. Uh...no.

Our decisions affected only the two of us 'till Spring 2005 when Maureen's stepfather died from a quick and aggressive form of pancreatic cancer. Before his passing, they had fortunately already made the trek back up near our home, but his condition kept them stuck in their motor home in Salem an hour south. We visited often of course, until, and through, his passing.

Maureen's mother had never driven the motor home, so Maureen's bus-driving experience proved valuable. The Elks Lodge had allowed her mother to stay parked at their site 'till Maureen could move her mother up with us. Maureen spent a lot of time with her mother going over personal items and taking care of all their affairs. In the end, I offered to let her come to live with us in the apartment they had finished in the basement. I invited her to stay with us as long as she needed, figuring once she had grieved a while and recovered her finances, she would assess where she wanted to live and find a place of her own.

We sold her mother's motor home, but not without difficulty. Her mother and stepfather had repeatedly traded up their motor homes in both size and amenities. They had kept rolling over the debt from the prior motor homes, so they were upside down in this last one. We finally sold it, but only by her mother adding money to get it gone. Several times, I heard from my mother-in-law how her husband would have "gotten more". I had long ago resigned myself to this fate as the disappointing son-in-law. If only I had become a doctor or lawyer.

All was not bad; I got promoted to a principal level in my design firm. Maureen showed me such support. However, it came with additional responsibilities and longer hours and travel. Maureen and I continued our commitment though, "if not working, then together." I often had two evening meetings a week and would travel overnight once or twice a month. I called frequently and rushed to see her, and she knew it. I would call the moment my plane landed (typically with a "hubba hubba"—our way of flirting) and stay on the phone, often until I walked in the door. I could drive from the airport to the house in twenty minutes.

These surprise rushes through the door made her giggle as I snuck in behind her while still talking on the phone. She would turn off the phone and smile, saying, "You goof." I would hold her so tightly each time. She loved that I always came home happy. I would rub her back and kiss her neck and explain that I had "touch deprivation". She would giggle again. I would then take her out for dinner. Just needing to feed the two of us, we had dinner whatever and whenever. We liked it that way.

We went everywhere together. Saturdays often included piled-up errands from the prior week. No matter if one had to rush into the post office, dash into the dry cleaner, or take a truckload to the dump, we instinctually did it together. "Oh the dump's great," she would claim. "You never know what you are going to see. If nothing else, it's great people watching." She made me laugh every time she went to the dump with me.

The grocery store might seem monotonous to some couples, and one could do it as easily as two, but we never thought twice about going together. We would grab some reusable bags, hold hands, find a cart, and I would push until we stopped at some aisle or the produce section. I would invariably stand behind her, take one finger to brush her hair from one side of her neck, and then place a light kiss near her ear with one hand on her waist. I would feel her smile as she bagged the broccoli. We did not just do this newly married. We did this every trip, every week, every year. We meant that much to each other.

We would walk on the waterfront or around the neighborhood and just hold hands instinctually. We had no problems with public displays of affection. Kissing her, hugging her, holding her hand, and often impromptu dancing near the Salmon Street fountains—all of it done effortlessly. We would say very little or talk endlessly about things to do. We acted on most of those ideas. Sometimes, though, the talks would be more serious.

"I don't want to be alone in my life again. I finally have something good. I told Candy that. I finally feel like I got it right," she confessed.

"I don't want you to ever have to be alone again either. I wish I could promise that," I said as it started to rain.

"Why can't you? Why can't you promise that?" she asked with a grin.

I laughed, "Well honey, a drunk driver could change everything. I cannot control that. I'm certainly not ever going to leave you on my own."

We walked on in the Portland drizzle, and she said nothing.

"Tell you what. I promise to live two weeks longer than you. I will stay with you through the end and take care of everything after. That should take about two weeks," I negotiated.

She laughed, "Sounds good."

We kissed on it.

Kisses in the rain.

Dancing in the rain.

This prompted me to get a life insurance policy, which made her feel more secure. Actually, it felt good to me too. I had not thought long-term before, but it made sense. I wanted her taken care of in case anything happened to me.

I had abandoned most of my friends and all my hobbies. Maureen retained a few good girlfriends from childhood, but life made their get-togethers infrequent. With your closest friends, you may not see each other for a year, yet when you do, you can fall right back into easy conversations. You always know how much you still mean to each other.

But for the entirety of our marriage, we preferred each other's company, and that made it a strong marriage—that and the ongoing open affection. We always kissed inside every single car wash. While checking the menus in restaurants, I would give her a large, exaggerated wink. She would laugh and give it right back.

We would delight in doing nothing together. Sometimes we just took a drive. We would go to downtown Portland and "drag the gut" as she called it: a throwback to the fifties. She had done it decades earlier with her first husband, but that memory had been stained by him angrily grabbing and dragging a stranger by his shirt collar for a block. The stranger had apparently said something derogatory, but Maureen had not heard it. She never understood her first husband's ongoing battles with anger.

Instead, she and I would just cruise slowly down Broadway Avenue, listen to music, and make better memories. We would especially run it at night to see the lit marquees as we rolled. It reminded her of her childhood, when her dad would drive up from Central Oregon to Portland and the lights would greet them from the Southwest Hills.

We would roll up Broadway with the windows rolled down. She would have the radio going. She loved music. With the music, though, came dance, and she married a guy with two left feet—me.

We would sway and do a modified two-step in the house or at a park all the time. We often had music playing, but Maureen wanted to go out dancing. Not being terribly graceful, I let my hesitation show. She knew she would have to convince me, but she had that superpower. Maureen just looked at me and said, "You know they have dance lessons. Dancing is very romantic." She then batted her eyes, knowing well how to motivate me. She also knew that I knew and what I would do. Of course, I found us dance lessons.

Arthur Murray seemed the right place to go, as I needed professional help.

We enrolled in the basic classes where they teach you the fundamentals. They break it down into six classic dances: Waltz, tango, foxtrot (slower tempo), and swing, rumba, and cha-cha (up-tempo). It took us a while to get the steps down, and for me to follow a rhythm. Maureen had great rhythm, as she had played the saxophone and piano earlier in life. She had the innate ability to just pick out a tune and sing it or play it by ear. She got that from her father and also instilled that in her son. I had no music on my side. I had a guitar I had given up on long ago. Still, dance made her happy, so very happy.

We would take weekly lessons and practice at home best we could, but then come back with questions about things we had forgotten.

> *I guide her hand to my waiting shoulder.*
> *Searching fingers caress my neck. We pose.*
> *Staring transfixed, I run my hand downward*
> *Finding the small dimple of her torso.*
> *Perfect. We let smiles curl our cheeks*
> *Breaking our frame, disregarding teacher.*
> *Joined for a kiss so light the wind could pass*
> *Between our lips but not steal our love.*
> *Your frame! Your frame! Respect the space! Again!*
> *And one, and two, and three, and four. We dance.*

We got better and built confidence. Maureen would continue to smile hours after each lesson. She would ask me in the car, "So did you enjoy it?"

I tried keeping my face straight and said, "No. I hated it." You get to a point in marriage where you can just feel your partner's smirk.

She poked me in the ribs and claimed victory, "You did too like it."

Laughing, I conceded, "Yes baby. I did. I like dancing with you." She would then cradle my arm.

To put the dancing into practice, Arthur Murray would have socials. She wanted to go to these until she found out that they like you to change up partners. She did not like that. She did not like that at all. We would deftly move and scurry and avoid awkward approaches so she could just keep dancing with me. She felt safe with me. She had built confidence in her own dancing and felt ok during the lesson with the instructor. Dancing with a stranger proved too hard for her though. The mental part got in the way, and she got flustered. Her smile left when she danced with other partners.

As time went on, we learned the basics of each dance. We felt confident to take the dancing to other venues. The company wanted us to sign up for more lessons and achieve a competition-level proficiency. Instead, we snuck away. We tried a couple of clubs but found much of the music geared toward people fifteen to twenty years our junior. Their dancing looked nothing like what we had learned. We then stumbled across the Baby Boomers Social Club. They played her kind of music. Everyone danced the same kinds of steps that we knew. Maureen had found her venue.

We went dancing there many weekends but preferred the first weekend of the month when the live bands played. The Grange Halls and Elks Clubs became our Saturday date nights. Those attending had various dancing proficiencies, from novice to well trained. Maureen had rocked to this music in her room as a teenager. They did mix in a few pop songs she heard now on the radio. I loved finding those opportunities, staying by her side and leading best I could. Those nights, her smile never stopped.

For nearly all our marriage, we danced.

Dancing proved a metaphor in our relationship as well. Maureen would lose confidence, and I would see it. I would respond with something to build that confidence back up just to watch it slip away in another direction. I kept weaving and bobbing, side to side. This dance, though, seemed to repair years of mental abuse or simply neglect. She would sometimes see it in herself too and join the dance.

This became an understood part of our routine. We would adjust when something made her sad. It might flare up as something that related to a childhood memory or memories of one of her earlier marriages or some other emotional pain. Together, we would build her confidence back up. She did not crumble; she cracked. She remained strong but weary. She remained happy but shaken. If you always keep your feet moving to the music, your heart and mind follow.

Speaking of music, Maureen listed concerts and musicals high on her list of priorities. She loved music with a passion and would recount some of her favorite childhood times rocking in her room in the sixties to Elvis, The Beatles, and The Beach Boys, and later to the Mamas and the Papas, Dylan, and The Stones. In 1976, on a fluke, a girlfriend invited her to go to an Elvis Presley concert in Eugene, Oregon on Thanksgiving Day. Eugene could get cold, so she kept her coat on. They had great seats (though they never sat). They were so close to the stage that as he started dabbing his brow and tossing those white scarves to the audience, she caught one and quickly tucked it under her coat. Other ladies clawed for it in vain. She kept it her whole life.

Maureen attended most of her concerts, though, after we got together. Whether in fancy music halls or outdoor venues on the grass, it never mattered. Whether part of a weekend lineup or a solo act, she loved it all. I could not help but indulge this vibrant, wide-eyed woman who just wanted to see, hear, and experience the fun things in life.

Some of Maureen's Favorite Concerts Over Our Twenty Years

The Rolling Stones	Paul McCartney	Ringo Starr	Paul Simon
Bruce Springsteen	Billy Joel	Elton John	Carlos Santana
Jim Brickman	Cher	Chicago	Cyndi Lauper
Stevie Wonder	Tim McGraw	John Mellencamp	Jewel
Carlene Carter	Josh Groban	The B-52's	The Gog-Go's
Hootie & The Blowfish	Huey Lewis & The News	Weird Al Yankovic	

We also supported a plethora of local Portland artists, particularly piano music. She enjoyed Michael Allen Harrison the most, especially his Christmas shows when Julianne Johnson, Haley Johnsen, and other incredible voices would come to the stage. We never missed a year. I would turn and watch her, whether at these concerts, some musical, or the symphony: she would sit mesmerized and so appreciative. She sometimes saw me looking at her out of the corner of her eye. Then she would grab my arm and smile. With a kiss, she would turn back again and watch the show unfold.

Maureen wanted to travel too. She had that dream as a little girl and kept it her whole life. That's what she journaled about the most. Her vacations up until the age of fifty had almost exclusively centered around camping. She had enjoyed camping initially, but after decades of setting up and striking camp sites, she had had enough.

On a walk we took along the Portland waterfront even before getting engaged, Maureen explained, "You need to understand something about me. You and I will NEVER go camping. I've done it, and I'm done."

As I had no particular propensity for camping, I agreed. For the next twenty years, roughing it meant downgrading to a four-star hotel. In fact, just a couple of years into our marriage, we got a time share in Mexico. She liked the idea of resorts and the ability to trade to other places around the globe.

We made a marriage pact: we promised each other to take a break from work and take at least two nice trips per year. We kept to that. One trip always included somewhere sunny and warm (when you live in Oregon, the winters can feel long). For the other trip we would just go somewhere of particular interest to her.

On our flights out, she liked to raise the armrest between the seats and cuddle. Sometimes I pretended mine did not work. "It won't raise up honey. It's broken."

I would receive one of those priceless smirks with one cocked eyebrow, "You're messing." She would raise the armrest and grab my arm and cuddle in for the flight. I loved those times.

On one of our earliest trips, we went to Kauai, which remained a favorite of hers forever. We first tried our hand at snorkeling on Kauai, and she marveled at the variety of fish off Poipu Beach. We also bought one of our first pieces of art. She never felt she had a voice before, but now had found it. She saw a pastel by Hale Pua and thought it was beautiful. That piece started our art collection, and we would acquire new art for years to come. She remembered that trip fondly, down to the silliest things. Our room did not come with a bottle opener, and we had bought some adult beverages. A local shop sold us a small wooden one, and we commented that it had "Aloha" on the side. The clerk corrected us, "Aloooo-ha." For years, we used that opener while saying, "Aloooo-ha."

She picked Sicily once—out of the blue. While we always tried to go to the local restaurants, she had a hard time skipping her Starbucks. I often scoped out the Starbucks nearest to our hotels for her. While I was planning our Sicily trip, I came across the fact that Italy had no Starbucks. When I shared this with Maureen, she almost changed destinations. I had to explain to my beautiful wife, "They have good coffee there too, baby. We will get by just fine." They did, and we did. However, the coffee proved too strong for her, and she downgraded to tea. It made us both laugh, though not as much as the fancy restaurant where we ordered a nice meal.

Apparently, we had not understood that the meal included lamb. She ate most of it, but not all. Her childhood demeanor kicked in, and she spat out a bit in her napkin. We thought nothing of it 'till the waiter came at the end to clear the table, and upon picking up the napkin, a large piece fell ("plop") right onto the table. He picked it up and whisked the plate away, but Maureen erupted in such a fit of embarrassed giggles that I could not help but join in.

In Paris, we decided to take the train to Versailles to see the palace. All recommendations were to get there early to avoid the long lines. I pleaded with Maureen to skip her Starbucks that morning, and she agreed. However, immediately after we got off the train, we saw a Starbucks between the station and the palace. I laughed and we looked at each other, and with a big kiss, I declared, "You win."

However, we almost didn't get to enter the palace. We waited at a side entrance as instructed while busloads of tourists lined up at the main entrance across the courtyard and down the block. The side entrance never opened, until a lone staff member came to the door and explained, "There is a worker strike today, so we are short-staffed. This entrance is closed today. You will have to go to the main entrance." She then closed the door again.

Now I had known Maureen to always behave in a reserved manner, but this just set her off. "This is ridiculous. We did what we were told," she said. I tried to calm her down and explained, "Yes, but honey with the strike…" I did not even get to finish. She walked briskly to the main entrance, skipping the line, and walked right up to the staff while asking me to flash our tickets. The woman asked, "Are you part of a group?" Maureen, without batting an eye, said, "Yes, this one right here going in now." They let us in. I should note that the group she claimed we belonged to all looked like teenage Asian students. We laughed about that for many years.

Our trips gave us countless fond memories. With me, Maureen found that she loved to travel. She saw her dreams come true and could hardly wait for the next trip. Often on our flights back, I would lean over and whisper, "Where to next, sweetheart?"

Our Tropical Trips

Kauai (twice)	Maui (twice)	Hawaii (Big Island)	Acapulco
Cancun (three times)	Los Cabos	Mazatlán (twice)	Puerto Vallarta (twice)
Saint Martin	Grand Bahamas	Barbados	

Our Other Destinations

England	Ireland	France	Sicily
Victoria B.C.	San Diego (twice)	Philadelphia	Niagara Falls
Washington D.C.	Orlando	Big Canoe, GA	New Orleans
New York City (twice)	Las Vegas (three times)	San Francisco (four times)	
Route 66	Disneyland, CA (ten times— she loved it)		

She appreciated everything. I realized that I had a rare find in this person so receptive to the world around her. However, with all that I tried to introduce her to, she thankfully changed my life far more.

I often had high energy. I was always planning, looking to move upward, finding the next opportunity, and selling the next project. I presented in front of a thousand people with the same confidence, intensity, and passion as when dealing with people one-on-one. I thought, "Make things happen."

Maureen loved to watch me. She saw the authenticity in it all. I never did show for show. I just ran to the next thing and the next. However, before Maureen, I never slowed down to savor it.

She accepted me for me but also showed me a way to temper my energy: to throttle it when the situation required. She did this by doing nothing else but staying calm. She would talk softly, and because I remained so smitten throughout our whole lives, I would quiet down. I would lean in and listen.

I had a career as a planner, but on our very first beach trip together back when we just started dating, she managed to slow me down. I had so many shops and restaurants and venues planned out. I remember we got there maybe an hour before sunset. On the Oregon coast, even in the summer, you often need a jacket. She threw one on and said, "Let's take a walk on the beach first before we go to dinner." She took my hand, and we stepped onto the sand.

As we walked, I continued to jabber on about twenty different things at once. She smiled and listened and walked. She then took more of my arm and leaned in with her head on my shoulder, and I stopped talking. It felt so good, warming me from the inside. The sun sat really low in the sky. She said, "Let's sit down."

I suggested, "There's a restaurant right up here. They have seats that look out right on the beach for the sunset."

"We are on the beach," she said. "The sunset's right here. Let's just sit here and watch it."

We did. We watched the sunset without any distractions and for no other purpose than to just watch it. This happened before everyone carried cameras in their phones. Hell, before everyone carried phones. We just watched it… together…holding each other while sitting on the sand. I had seen countless sunsets before of course, but never really just looked at one and quieted myself and took it in.

We watched the sky turn from blue to yellow to orange to red to purple as the sun touched down in the Pacific. In the dim light she asked me, "Doesn't the tide sound strong? It crashes but calms you too. Isn't that funny?"

I listened. I could hear a few people around us here and there; a dog barking, kids laughing, moms collecting the day's paraphernalia, and small groups starting fires on the beach with the first crackles of the flames. One-by-one I silenced each of them and focused on the waves. That rhythm of crash and roll and recede overlapped with a wave behind it, and another behind that. You can hear each of them: crash, roll, recede. All my times at the beach before, I had kept myself busy, and the tide was merely background noise. Now Maureen helped me make the tide the focus. I had this beautiful woman next to me showing a man in his thirties the beach like it was his first time. Surely nobody ever provided love with such quiet grace.

> *"...I love thee to the depth and breadth and height*
> *My soul can reach, when feeling out of sight*
> *For the ends of being and ideal grace.*
> *I love thee to the level of every day's*
> *Most quiet need, by sun and candle-light..."*
> *Elizabeth Barrett Browning, Sonnet 43*

Maureen gave me that gift—her strength, which became mine too, to sit still and listen.

Her demeanor from that day throughout all the years of our marriage never failed to bring me back to my center. However, a calm and quiet demeanor did not mean that she did not still dream big. Little did I know, five years into our marriage, that she had her heart set on our next adventure: building a new home.

Chapter 5

Our Home

*I*n the Fall of 2005, Maureen drove a particular bus route that took her up on the east hills and by the Willamette National Cemetery. There lay her uncle (a veteran) and aunt who had passed just a few years prior. Maureen was always diligent about placing flowers on their grave.

Near the top of the hill, she saw this sign for an undeveloped residential parcel. From the time she started that route, the sign read "Sale Pending". After work I would hear about this amazing site, but a sale remained pending. As such, it never went beyond the occasional mention. This all changed one September day when she came home elated with the news, "The site is available. We can buy it."

I looked at her, not sure I had all the pieces. "You mean the site up on the hill?"

"Yes. I was driving by today and took a look at the sign and the 'pending' part was gone. I stopped the bus and got one of the flyers."

"Honey. Were there people on the bus?" I asked.

"Oh yeah, but they didn't mind." I loved my wife and chuckled at that thought. I started to look for something to make dinner. I turned back to give her options. She stared at me, stunned. "We have to go!"

"What, now?"

"Yes, or somebody else will get it. Get your coat."

I apparently had no idea how much this site had occupied her thoughts.

We got in the car and drove up. The site was about twenty minutes away. I had heard about this infamous site, but because it had a sale pending, had thought nothing of it. That proved my mistake.

We got to the turnoff. "There!! There!!" she exclaimed.

"Honey, this is a private gravel drive."

"Yes. Pull over in that wide spot," she explained.

I stared at two homes over the steering wheel: one from the sixties and one brand new. The new one had a simple split-level design, but I thought it might have a nice view. As I got out of the car, I saw a trike in the front yard. I said, "Honey, it looks like it is sold, and somebody already moved in."

"No, not the house, the site down there," she said and pointed.

I then noticed the small for sale sign pointing down a hillside between the two homes. Not yet dusk, we made our way down the hill overgrown with brush and blackberry bushes. We got to the end of the fence line and saw the lot. Some tires, cans of mystery fluid, and a crushed mailbox sat abandoned at the bottom of the hill. Blackberry bushes at least a dozen feet tall covered much of the property. A few trees and a lot of brush covered the rest. The whole thing sloped at least at a 15% grade down to what appeared to be a creek and a more heavily wooded area. I had a hard time telling where the site stopped and some sort of common creek or greenbelt started. I saw no evidence of any utilities. The grade worried me a lot, along with the environmental and potential wetland issues. At that point, I had spent seventeen years in the planning, design, and construction business, and my head swirled with a dozen reasons to run from this site.

Maureen came down behind me. I turned around towards her. She stood there beaming like she had found gold. She squealed, "What do you think?"

In that instant, I thought about the house she had wanted to get in her first marriage, and how she got outvoted. I thought of the trips she wanted to go on before we had met, the dreams she wanted to pursue but was never supported in by family, and the life she had wanted but was only starting to get a taste of now. I thought how often someone in her life told her no: likely for far fewer reasons than all the ones I saw before us now.

I could say only one thing to this woman that I married five years prior and still remained utterly smitten with, "It'll be perfect dear. This is a great find."

We took that walk on Thursday night. By Sunday, we owned the site.

We spent a year designing our house. We scoured the area for sales on plumbing and lighting fixtures and would store them for the eventual build. We looked at paints and tiles and marble. Maureen liked aspects of Victorian homes, so we scoured old plans and photos where we grabbed a bit of this and a bit of that. Maureen loved the Victorian era.

We did not design the house as an authentic Victorian but included many similar traits—the traits she liked. Over the months as I drew the plans, she would lean over my shoulder and ask questions, "Where's the butler pantry?"

"For the butler we don't have?" I teased.

"Every Victorian home had a butler pantry," she replied. I added a butler pantry between the kitchen and dining room.

I would draw more, and she would come back again, "Where's the nursery?" This question alarmed me far more. I turned with a surprised look.

She smiled, knowing me all too well at this point, "No dear: that ship has sailed. But every Victorian home had a nursery." She was thinking of her son starting his family and coming to visit. I added a nursery with a pocket door off one of the guest bedrooms.

We collaborated on nearly all of the design, at least the parts she cared about. Fearing that her mother would live with us for a while, but probably not forever, we created a bedroom, bathroom, and den on the main floor that she could have for her private use. Hard of hearing, her mother would often turn the TV up really loud. As such, I had the walls and ceiling of the den insulated.

We cut the garage into the hillside. Rains created several mudslides in the region due to poor engineering. We avoided stilts.

To get a sense of height, I took two fourteen-foot two-by-fours, attached them together, and placed a camcorder at the end (olden days). I hit record to see what I would see that far up. We could have a view, but several trees stood in the way. If we wanted the view back to downtown Portland, we would have to get over the trees. The film pointed to the fact that we needed a loft above the second floor. We had already drawn a garage level plus two floors.

We made the loft big enough for our master bedroom, a bathroom, and our walk-in closet. We also included a small, round, covered deck off our bedroom, equipped with a weathervane. It had a similar feel to the Victorian cupolas but without the gingerbread. Neighbors called it our floating gazebo. Based on the gymnastics I made our structural engineer go through, that proved an appropriate description. We designed it big enough for two chairs and a small bistro table… and a bottle of wine. It overlooked the trees to downtown and the sunset.

We had done a bit of antiquing in our early marriage, so this new Victorian-ish home provided a chance to do more. Maureen wanted an old mantel for the fireplace. We installed a fireplace in her mother's den too. We scored two of them, both removed from early 1900 homes: one from Portland, and one salvaged from a home in New Orleans after Katrina.

For the crowning touch, Maureen wanted a real crystal chandelier in the dining room. When we saw the price tags, I explained the illegal activities I would have to partake in to afford such a fancy light to Maureen. She let me off the hook, and we continued to shop. We ended up at a reclaimed lighting store where crystal chandeliers hung next to turning disco balls and art deco lamps. We found a salvaged chandelier with real crystal in wonderful shape and a tenth the cost of new. We snatched it up. Considering the bargain, she picked out two more for the foyer and the landing in front of our bedroom.

We secured a contractor but found the price exceeding our budget. We decided to cut back on some things that we ended up doing ourselves. The contractor started late in October 2006. We put our then-current home on the market, not knowing how long it would take to sell. It sold in less than thirty days. We had to move to a two-bedroom apartment with us, her mother, and five cats.

During that year of building, we defined the phrase "labor of love."

To keep costs down, we pulled a lot of things out of the contractor's scope to buy and install ourselves. The house had grown to a 4,200 square foot living area, a three-car garage, plus over 1,200 square feet of deck on a 0.6-acre site. Maureen had always dreamed of an old classic home where both of her kids and all her grandkids could come to visit for the holidays and everyone have a place to sleep. She got that, and it served that purpose for several years. She loved family and wanted to create a warm and comfortable place for the growing grandkids to call "Grandma's house". She spent a lot of time actively healing relationships and wanted somewhere for everyone to feel at home.

As part of the construction, Maureen and I primed and painted the whole interior. We stained, varnished, and trimmed all thirty-six doors and forty-two windows. We pre-purchased and direct-hired all the flooring. It was a mix of teak, bamboo, and carpet. We purchased and installed all the cabinetry.

We purchased some marble tops and made others out of tile. Tiles were factory seconds out of a sense of sustainability. However, Maureen wanted nice marble. Neither of us had ever gone into a slab warehouse to pick marble out before, and we had no idea what to expect. Down each aisle we went, with a couple catching her eye, but not until the last aisle in the far back corner, literally the last slab, did she say, "This one is beautiful." As fate would have it, that one had no price tag on it. I trekked back to the front office and explained this "blue one" we had seen. They smiled, "Oh, THAT one." I had hoped for a different response. I have explained that I never told my wife "no". This brought me about as close as I ever got. We compromised and did this blue granite in one bathroom and a similar (less expensive) veining marble with a chocolate color in most other areas. She liked the choices.

Lastly, we purchased and planted one hundred and thirty-five native trees and bushes as a condition of the permit. Of course, we had a heat wave, and the plants started dying before we could get them planted. We set them in the creek, dug holes, ran down to the creek, grabbed two at a time, and brought them back up to plant—back and forth. It left us exhausted. Later, we added more ornamentals, including many roses. She had her fragrant favorites—Double Delight and Love's Promise.

A month before we planned to move in, we toured her best friend Candy and her husband John through the nearly finished home. Our contractor had not yet laid the carpet, but they had textured the walls. Maureen and I had also already primed and painted all the walls and ceilings. It was a Saturday night, and we had set out to grab dinner together when as we headed out, we heard a faint, "meow".

We had told the workers to close the doors at the end of each day to avoid getting strays in the house since we now had the finishes in place. We searched all over for that cat. As improbable as it seemed, the cry came from the second-floor ceiling joists. Access hatches did not reach this space.

Maureen and I looked at each other, and we knew we really had no choice. I grabbed a hammer and knocked a big hole in the newly finished ceiling, reached up, and pulled out a recently born kitten. I thought, "How is this possible?" I shined the flashlight forward in the joist bay and saw no other cats. This one's eyes still remained mostly shut.

Given it was a Saturday night, we took it to the emergency vet. They refused to take it unless we wanted it put down. They said they needed the mom to nurse it. Alternatively, we could take it home and bottle-feed it. True friends, Candy and John offered to bottle feed the kitten 'till we found the mother cat. I had no idea how to go about that.

Sunday, Maureen and I continued working in the house on that same floor, when late in the morning, we heard a thud. I walked back around the corner and found a kitten on the floor below the hole. I had checked before. I had seen no more kittens. Where did this one come from? We imposed on our friends, "Since you're feeding one, do you want to feed two? We will find the mother." They obliged.

Sunday night, no mother cat. Monday morning, Maureen went back to work, but I took a few days off to get the tiling done. I was working in the top loft setting the shower tile. When I turned for a tool, I saw a kitten staring at me. "Meow?" What in the world?! I then understood that the mother cat must have come all the way up to the loft and had the litter under our bathtub through the side access door. I saw the plumbers had overcut the hole in the floor for the drainpipe, so kittens one and two, blind, wandered until they fell through into the ceiling cavity below. This third one had avoided that fall and came toward me where it heard the noise. I had to alternate between setting tile and bottle-feeding for the day 'till Maureen got off work. When all the other workers left, we waited quietly in the loft bathroom.

Sure enough, when the site went quiet, the mother cat came up the stairs to look for her litter. I waited quietly in that bathroom, hidden, thinking I would shut the door and catch her once she got inside. I stood in the shower and waited. She crept in. I tried to get to the door, but she saw me and darted out.

Fortunately, she became desperate to see her kittens, so I waited, and she returned. This time I shut the door and trapped her. This did not make her happy. She meowed and hissed and ran around. I finally calmed her down. I pet her a lot and gave her some food. She let me pick her up. Maureen had the third kitten (I checked— there were no others).

We carefully introduced kitten to mother, and they bonded. We picked up the other two kittens from our amazing friends, and kept the mother and kittens in the downstairs garage storage room for four weeks. We fed and petted them and took care of the litter box while our five cats occupied the room next to them. We knew we could not keep nine cats. No matter the humor of the story, we had to find homes for the four new ones. We did. In fact, our friends took back the ones they had bottle-fed and named them Lewis and Clark.

We put a lot into that home while working full-time jobs. We had several tired moments and a lot of laughable ones, but we never had one fight. We danced in each room whether finished or not. Love does that to you. This house fulfilled a dream of Maureen's, and I lived my dream each day, married to this person who accepted me so unconditionally.

We moved into our new home on October 5, 2007 and would know nearly eleven years in that house together. We had expected many more. I can look back and feel thankful that we kept going and doing while we could. Maureen did not just enjoy travel and music, but watching sports as well: especially live and in person.

We had our local Oregon favorites, like the Portland Trailblazers, and we saw four or five games per year. She would often indulge me as I painted my face. "Not on me," she declared. We would venture up to Seattle to catch a Seahawks game and made a trip of it. Among all of these, we had one very memorable sports trip.

We liked our Oregon Ducks college football team, and they did very well in their 2014 season. So well, in fact, that the NCAA named them as one of the four teams to make it to the first-ever college championships. I recall reading the official announcement in early December.

As we did in the morning almost every weekend, I made Maureen's coffee (two sugars) and brought it to her while she sat in her robe. I then got the paper and my coffee. I would separate the sections she liked from the sections I liked. Oddly, we liked completely different parts of the paper, but we read things to each other that we thought the other would like.

I read to her, "Well honey, it's official, the Ducks are in the championships. They play Florida State in the Rose Bowl, New Year's Day in Pasadena."

"That's good," she replied with her nose well into the front page.

Several minutes passed 'till she said, "We should go to one of those things."

I had moved on to other stories, "What thing baby?"

"One of those bowl thingies," she absently suggested. She liked watching sports but did not always have the vernacular down. I loved her.

"You mean the Rose Bowl?"

"Yeah. That Marcus Mariota seems like a very polite young man," she said, now thumbing the *Parade Magazine* insert.

I thought, "Ok. That's as good a reason as any."

"Are you serious?!" I asked. "I mean, that is great, but the game is less than a month away. I have to get tickets this morning, flights, hotels...you know," I stammered.

"Ok," she softly replied as she read about the health dangers of white bread.

I leapt into action on the computer and first looked for game tickets. Seeing the price, I considered going to an alternate site to sell a kidney, but instead I stayed the course. Game tickets—check. Hotel in the general proximity—check. Flights—allowing an extra day for sightseeing—check. Car as an add-on—check. She would want to see the Rose Parade ahead of the game, so we needed some reserved seats—check. We would fly in the night before (New Year's Eve), so she would want to go dancing. Find a venue and get tickets with a dinner—check.

Pleased with my accomplishments, I grabbed us both another cup of coffee and sat back down in the front room triumphantly. She was still reading the paper.

"Well, I did it. We're going to Pasadena."

Without looking up, she said, "Thank you baby. They have a sale at Macy's we should go to." She had made it to the Christmas ads.

Again, we enjoyed and lived this life: she had the vision, and I executed the plan.

As such, I have asked myself this question dozens of times: did that approach to our marriage mask the early signs of

Frontotemporal Degeneration (FTD)? Did she have it earlier than we started noticing it? It seemed like it would have showed up at work, but it did not. Perhaps the type of work hid the symptoms from us. She had no need for learning new technologies, and I did all the planning. As such, perhaps the FTD stayed hidden.

Maureen had not spent much time in a modern office or workplace. As with most of us, she had multiple odd jobs throughout life, including waitressing and retail. She had performed a little office work in the seventies and eighties and into the early nineties, but only sporadically. The world had not moved to computers at that time. We had hard copies and typewriters (ask your grandparents to explain).

She spent most of her career driving buses. That work has many technical challenges, but driving also becomes an almost instinctual habit in a different part of the brain. It included detailed work: learning new routes, maintaining schedules, and updating safety training on ever-changing bus types. There was a complexity to it that would surely have made the FTD reveal itself, if she had it.

The world, though, developed technology around her, so she never had a reason to learn how to use it. She had little need for email or internet searches. She never developed an interest in social media, but would rather just call her friends. When asked to pay bills online, plan a trip using the internet, or keep up with her grandson's girlfriend's status on Facebook, she found it confusing.

We had all gone through the evolution of the bricks to the flip phones to the stylus instruments and then the touch screens. We experienced the progression, and she did not. Technology never held any importance for her. Without the need to learn new technology, did I miss her early FTD cues? I do not think so. No other aspect of her life seemed affected. Although she did get to a point where she wanted to look into early retirement.

In early 2013, she came to me and asked, "Do you think it's possible for me to retire?" Changes at her job put in place by administrators had riled the community and the riders. Sadly, the more disgruntled riders took it out on the drivers with some being spat on, hit, and verbally abused. The drivers did nothing wrong: they just worked on the front line.

Maureen had not experienced this abuse firsthand, but drivers in the break area had growing concerns and complaints. It made the whole thing unpleasant.

With me at forty-five and her at sixty-two, I had not given any thought yet to retirement, but I should have. I could see she started to become unhappy, so I committed myself to getting her retired. We would work on it together. We had built our beautiful home, and the mortgage remained steep. While it would have paid better to wait 'till she was sixty-six, she needed relief. I could see it in her eyes.

She had social security and a couple of pensions she could tap. Her pensions included the school district and the city bus system. I could slice it multiple ways.

Many years earlier, we had taken out life insurance policies: a very modest one on her, but a large one on me, as I wanted her taken care of should something happen. Our plans for retirement needed to echo this strategy. I knew that because I travelled so much, I had an increased risk of a drunk driver leaving her a widow.

We maximized the benefits, which meant sacrificing the survivor portion. If she passed before me, it would leave nothing for me. I knew though, that if something happened to me, with the life insurance and 401K, she could sell the home, pay cash for a small place near her kids, and still have plenty of money left in the bank. She would also have an ample monthly income from her retirement. It seemed like the right plan, so we made it happen. She retired the day after her sixty-third birthday.

That last day of work, she drove an afternoon route that ended on the road and meeting a relief driver. I had taken the afternoon off and created a giant banner. As she pulled up to the stop, she saw me holding this huge banner saying "Congratulations Maureen!! You Did it!! Happy Retirement!!" Of course, I held flowers in one hand as well.

The passengers talked amongst themselves. The relief driver looked at me and asked Maureen about it. She confirmed it, turned to the bus, and said with a huge smile, "My last day!" They clapped for her. She stepped off the bus, came over to me, and said in her typical way, "You goof." With a big hug and kiss, I whisked her off to happier days.

Soon after, with her newfound time, I arranged piano lessons for her. A teacher would come to our home once a week and give her lessons. This thrilled Maureen. She had played the piano off and on in her life with some lessons in her childhood, but had fallen out of it. We had a beautiful 1917 H.L. Phillips upright in the front room that she had found in the paper years earlier. We had designed the front room with space on an inside wall to keep it in tune. She excelled, and the teacher (half Maureen's age) thoroughly enjoyed the variety Maureen wanted to play, from classic rock to modern showtunes (she had a thing for the *Gladiator* theme). She also enjoyed playing gospel.

It seemed retirement would work out well. However, it started a bit rocky, with her mother still living with us for over eight years by then. With retirement came more time at home with her mother. The little things, often unnoticed or tolerated, now became more difficult. Maureen remained silent but I knew she was frustrated.

While certainly a good person, her mother was very particular about the way she liked things. Now with Maureen retired and home more, she did more around the house. This became a problem. Maureen would move things, and her mother would move them back. Maureen would rearrange things, and her mother would criticize it and wanted it back the way she had it. Maureen would leave a glass or newspaper out, and her mother would walk behind her and put it away, causing Maureen to later search for it. Maureen would play the piano, and her mother would call from the next room, "Sounds pretty good, but still making a few mistakes."

Her mother wanted to go for a coffee with Maureen most days, and when Maureen wanted to run errands instead, her mother insisted on coming too. Maureen sometimes just needed that time alone to get things done. Maureen had no understanding of how to tell her mother no. She never learned that in sixty-four years.

She loved her mother immensely, but we had spent nine years under the same roof. For eight of those, Maureen and I had worked, so we led our lives and her mother hers. Maureen had gone from seeing her mother in the evenings and weekends at home to now nearly every waking moment of every day. She felt trapped, criticized, and controlled. Self-doubt started to creep back in.

After a year of this, I came home one evening to find Maureen hiding upstairs in our bedroom. I asked why, and she said her mother could not come up there because of her bad knee. Maureen simply needed some space. I saw that she was physically shook and withdrawn. I pleaded, "Talk to me."

"I'm living in my mother's house," she said.

"No, honey, this is your house," I consoled.

She said no, and explained everything that had gone on every day for the first year of her retirement. She said each thing seemed small and trivial, but so many little things every single day had just started to take their toll. She felt like that little girl again, always being corrected.

I did not want my wife's golden years spent feeling like she could not do what she wanted to in her own home. I didn't want her to feel criticized or controlled. I knew that, at sixty-four, she could not suddenly stand up to her mother.

I asked, "Do you want me to find her her own place? It has been over nine years. She should have found a place by now. We didn't push, so it never happened."

She got teary. "I don't want to hurt Mom, but I can't keep living like this."

I played the heavy. My love for Maureen made her all things to me.

I went to the den to speak with her mother. Paper and pen in hand, I asked her how the years of apartment hunting had gone. She said she had looked but found nothing fitting her needs. I asked what "looked" meant. I ferreted out that once or twice a year, she did drive-bys of facilities, grabbed a flyer, or talked to a friend on the phone. She would find a place too expensive and would stop looking. She did not know computers and the internet, so I don't blame her, but the process seemed doomed to never get done.

I asked her what she wanted in a place, and she told me every-thing, including cost, amenities, location, etc. In two weeks, I found a place matching all the criteria and showed it to Maureen first. She liked it for her mother. She liked it a lot. We brought her mother there, and she did not take it well. What she could find fault with, she did. She also felt like we had kicked her out. We had taken her in when her husband died and said she could stay as long as she needed to. She had heard, "as long as she wanted to," not "needed to". She had also never learned to budget or save money very well, so our plan was flawed. She had lived with us in the old house for eighteen months, then the apartment for a year while the new house got built, and then in the new house for seven years. She got comfortable, and we ignored it. We admitted as much fault on our part as hers. We moved her out late 2014.

We tried to explain to her mother that she would be with people her own age and would meet lots of friends. She said she would not. However, inside of a month, she had a circle of at least six friends. Maureen still took her mother out once a week for coffee or vice versa. Their relationship grew stronger, and Maureen grew happier. She could flourish in her retirement again.

We continued to travel. Maureen also came with me on business trips – some good, some boring, but we loved our time together. After school board meetings, she would sometimes ask me, "Do you like those meetings?"

"No, they are just necessary for the job."

"Good," she would say, "because they are so boring." We would laugh. "Yes," I told her, "I assume the same sentiment is held by many Board members." You almost wished for a controversy to liven things up.

Maureen continued the piano. I convinced her to make her crafts and greeting cards again. I asked her if she wanted to pursue her dream of a real estate license, but she decided that window had closed.

She tended to her garden and planted wonderful flowers and vegetables, and I could hear her sing as she did this. She hung pots and drew in the hummingbirds that she delighted in. She loved the scent of flowers. I remember her smell:

> She smelled like a garden just after a light spring rain. The earth releases a fresh smell and a warmth as the sun soaks back up the rain. There are wildflower smells about the earth, like if you lay among the flowers and breathed in the lavender and lilacs, and even hints of vanilla, all among the deep, rich soil. That warm and fresh renewal—that was her scent.

All seemed well 'till Spring Break 2016, when everything started unraveling.

Chapter 6

Our New Reality

Maureen's son had asked her to come down and watch the girls as he had to work and needed a sitter for part of the spring break week. She of course came down to spend time with her latest two granddaughters, now nine and seven. They had activities to get to. Maureen got a bit confused. I had to stay behind and work. I had heard about a little confusion with their schedules but thought nothing of it. I thought she had just gotten a little rattled by the pace and busyness. We led a calm life, not that structured.

Kissing her son and grandchildren goodbye, she drove away to come back home to me. She got lost—lost in a town she had lived in for many years. She called me at work in the morning after she left her son's house. She had gotten turned around and was not sure how to get on the freeway. She had trouble reading the signs and interpreting what they said. She called me while driving, and I begged her to pull over in a parking lot. She did.

I slowly walked her through reading the signs. I tried to figure out where she was parked first. I asked her if she wanted to stay there, and I would drive down (two hours). She said, "No. I just got confused. If I can get on the freeway, I will be fine."

I figured out where she parked and then talked her back on the road and to the needed turns. She got on the freeway. She just had to go straight for ninety-five miles, take our normal turnoff, and twenty minutes later she would be home. I convinced myself that she just had a misstep and would make it home safely. We would sort it out that afternoon.

Two hours later, she called my office rather than my mobile and spoke to the receptionist. Maureen did not know where she had ended up. She had driven to an unfamiliar part of town, as she had missed the normal turnoff and ended up in west Portland. The receptionist lived in the neighborhood and talked her back on the road to familiar settings and home.

I left work early and went to her. I hugged her. She was very shaken by the ordeal, and we walked through it together. Her son called and said she had struggled to be on time for activities, and that the girls had arrived a little late to some of them. This bothered Maureen; the fact that he would call and "tell on her," as she put it. I told her son to just back off and let us assess. Maureen felt embarrassed. This had all come on so suddenly. We had no advance warning; nothing. I worried what had just happened to my baby.

I consoled her (and myself) by thinking that maybe being so relaxed in retirement and our casual lives and then being thrown back into the stress of a rigid schedule had just messed with her sense of logic. However, I watched that next thirty days to try and pick up on things. Dementia never entered my mind, even over the course of that month when things unraveled further.

She seemed to be back to normal behavior. She drove to the store and ran limited errands, and all seemed fine in those respects.

However, I started to see little things around the house: clothes in the washer but not turned on; water brewed in the coffee pot but no coffee in the filter; things left out on the counters like half-eaten yogurts.

When we did the dishes together, I would rinse and hand them to her, and she would put them in the dishwasher. But then, the third or fourth dish in, she would dry it and put it in the cupboard. I explained, "Honey, I haven't washed those yet. They need to go in the dishwasher."

She would go, "Oh", take it out, and put it in the dishwasher. No sense of embarrassment, just a course correction.

Maureen loved to swim and asked for a pool. We put in a twenty-four foot diameter, above-ground pool cut into the hillside, so the half closest to the house sat flush with the grade. We could not afford an in-ground pool, but this would still work well. The plan was to build a wooden deck that would abut.

I hired out the digging after a failed personal attempt to operate a small backhoe on mud and a slope. I tipped it (stupid). I set the bottom ring and enlisted Maureen's help to steady the steel walls as I unrolled it and set it in the small track. With sand spread, I stood on a ladder on the inside, but I had neglected to bring a chair over on the outside to step down on (the walls were a little over four feet tall). Maureen stood looking at the various pieces—studying them.

"Honey. Can you bring the chair over to me?" I asked.

"Yeah," she said. She turned to look at the chair, saw a pair of my work gloves on it, and froze.

"Honey? The chair?"

She stared at the chair, and I watched the gears turn in her head. After a bit of this, I could see things simply not firing. Calmly, I said, "Sweetheart. Please pick up the gloves."

She did.

"Now put the gloves on the ground."

She did.

"Now pick up the chair and bring it to me."

She did.

My heart sank as I saw this unfold. I stepped out of the pool, thanked her, and gave her a hug. A big lump welled up in my throat.

During those weeks in April, I could see she kept thinking about these issues. I would come home and find her sitting in the same spot in the front room day after day. I would call her multiple times per day as I always did. She would talk on the phone with me but speak less, with shorter answers.

She would be more elated than usual when I got home. She always wanted to go out and eat. She liked to go out at the end of each day. She slowly continued to pull away from actively doing things around the house.

Four weeks after the driving issue and the myriad of little things at home, I sat her down.

"Baby. I have been noticing some things lately. It seems like you are a little off. Are you ok?" I asked.

"Yeah," she replied, but she looked down.

"Do you see some things in yourself that don't seem right?"

"I guess so. I get confused. I don't use right words," she stammered out a confession. "But I'm ok."

I hugged her. "Sweetheart, you probably are ok, but it seems like it makes you sad. You seem like you do not do things you used to do. You do not even talk much anymore. Are you happy?"

"Yeah..." she trailed off unconvincingly while still holding me.

"What would you say to seeing the doctor?"

"I don't know if they can do anything," she pushed back.

"Well maybe not, but maybe they can," I tried to reason. "Maybe they can do some bloodwork. Maybe it is just a vitamin deficiency. Maybe you just need to be eating more of a kind of food or we get you a vitamin or something." Again, dementia had not entered my mind, but I knew this had grown into a big deal. I tried to downplay it so she would go to the doctor, because I had no idea what else to do.

"I guess so," she said.

"I promise. We will figure out what this is. We will deal with it. Ok? It's probably no big deal," I said as I prayed inside.

We went to her primary care doctor, and in the exam room they asked the standard security question, "Date of birth?"

The nurse waited. "Can you tell me your birthday?"

Maureen sat silently, but her eyes were actively searching for the answer.

I asked, "Honey. Can you tell the nurse your birthday?" while holding Maureen's hand.

She looked at me, trying to form the words, but no sound came out.

"It's..." I mouthed the word April to get her to say it with me.

"April. Yeah," she repeated.

"What's the day, honey? I am sorry, the date. Your birthday," I coached.

"April...twenty..." she struggled. More than being a memory issue, it seemed she could not form the words.

"Seven..." I softly finished.

"Twenty-seven," she said and smiled.

I turned to the nurse and said, "1950."

Afterward, they took her blood pressure and temperature but found nothing negative. The nurse left, and we waited for the doctor. I held Maureen's hand and kissed her on the cheek. This was starting to look worse than I thought. I guess I had not asked her to recall anything recently. We just sort of lived in the moment. We held hands. We kissed. We went out shopping, or to the movies, or dancing. I paid bills and took care of the mundane tasks behind the scenes. The two worlds of technical tasks and fun never much intersected for her. Now we were sitting there and she couldn't say her birthday.

Similar conversations occurred with her doctor, and while she ordered a blood test, she also made a referral for an MRI of Maureen's brain to "rule things out."

I kept reassuring Maureen. I made the test appointments. To be in a town with access to multiple clinics proved a blessing. I could push for earlier dates even if we had to go to different places. I explained to my employer that I would need to be out periodically to take my wife to these tests. They understood. As a principal in the firm, I had always shown dedication and worked long hours. They could flex, I thought. I designated some staff to cover meetings for me when a conflict arose.

I quietly explained these mental clarity issues to Maureen's piano teacher. Her teacher said that she had noticed a decline in the last four to six weeks. Maureen hadn't been catching on to the new music as she used to, and she wanted to play the same couple of tunes over and over again. She asked if we should take a break from the lessons. I said no. I knew that Maureen looked forward to them, and they gave her joy.

I found that the tests, which also included some in-clinic association tasks, were weighing heavily on both her and I. I thought about this all the time. I sat in my car and wondered what had happened, each week fearing a worse condition than the week before.

But I dumped my worries at the door. I would come in, smile, and give her big hugs and kisses, and she would just light up—my baby, my everything. I would have songs she knew on my phone and hit play or come in with them playing already. Then I'd take her by the hand and dance with her there in the front room. She would giggle and always oblige a dance offered. She would look at me, so in love, and me back at her the same way.

I would ask her how her day went, but found that she struggled to answer. She had trouble conveying a narrative. I changed to more pointed questions, "Did you eat today? Did you pet the cats? Did you read your magazines? Did you water your flowers? Did you play your piano? Did you talk to anyone on the phone?" I tried to mine for details of how she spent her day when I had to work.

A neurologist had looked at her MRI and suggested some follow up in-clinic tests, but we arranged to have someone come to the house and do tests as well. They would have her hold on to the worker's hands and pull on them to test strength and differences in one side or the other. They would have her hold things to test for shakes. Those went well. They would say three words to Maureen and ask her to repeat them back. Those did not go so well. They gave her a piece of paper and pencil and asked her to draw a circle. She struggled but eventually got an oblong drawn.

"Good," the worker said at our dining room table, "Now, I want you to write numbers in it like the face of a clock." Maureen froze up.

I coached, "Honey, like a clock, she wants you to put in the twelve numbers. Can you start with one? Put the one where it goes like on a clock."

She struggled, and then drew a one around the 3:00 position. "And now a two," I said. She drew the two in about the five position, and running out of room on the circle after six, she then skipped ahead and put the twelve at the top. I felt empty inside watching this unfold. I looked at my beloved and felt like something had simply stolen her mind. "No," I thought. She had her mind. I could see it searching for answers, but not able to produce them. I saw it all there in her eyes, but something kept her from understanding basic ideas. I felt tremendous sadness.

"Can you draw clock hands to show me 2:00?" the worker half-heartedly asked my wife.

Maureen put the pencil down. She felt overwhelmed—done. She took my hand from my lap and looked at me. She felt sad too.

I could not coach her out of this and convince her she had done ok. She knew she had not.

Toward the end of June, we had our last visit with the neurologist. She had previously mentioned some irregularities in the MRI. Maureen had undergone multiple cognitive tests. Bloodwork showed nothing. I drove her to our normal hospital and sat waiting for the neurologist. Maureen sat quietly. I hugged her, held her hand, and kissed her multiple times on the temple, assuring her that no matter what, I would help her with whatever was wrong.

They showed us in and we exchanged pleasantries.

The neurologist then said very calmly, "I am sorry, but I am very confident that Maureen, you have what they call Frontotemporal Degeneration—FTD. It is a form of dementia."

We sat stunned. I held Maureen's hand and could feel it tighten.

I asked, "Dementia? Other than a brief bout of dementia at the end of her aunt's life, her family does not have a history of that. Right honey?" Maureen shook her head no. "Are you sure?" I asked the doctor.

"Yes. I am familiar with FTD, and the MRI confirms atrophy in the frontal lobe with some in the temporal region as well. The prior cognitive tests we did together in-clinic and the other tests ran at your home ruled out many other types and seem to confirm this. There is not a lot of exposure to it here among our staff. It is somewhat rare compared to something like Alzheimer's."

She continued, "FTD is not necessarily hereditary. It can be. It is not a memory issue like Alzheimer's but can be a symptom later in the disease." She turned toward Maureen and said, "You have the language side of this, I think—Primary Progressive Aphasia. There is also a behavioral side. That is not to say that the symptoms are exclusive." The neurologist allowed a long pause for us to digest this—me holding Maureen's hand and stroking her arm.

I stammered, "What are the next steps? What do we do?"

"We will want to do a few more confirming cognitive tests to understand the severity and the major symptoms as a baseline. We will also want to work with a speech pathologist to help maintain some verbal skills in the short term. There are several things we can try to help manage the symptoms, but there is not a cure."

"But," I interrupted, trying to find answers, "I mean it is just something we live with that we adjust for, right?"

The doctor stared right at both of us. "I'm sorry, but no. It will get worse. Most dementia proves eventually fatal. People with FTD have an expected lifespan of seven to ten years."

Maureen's grip gave way.

While the news of dementia can devastate a family, as it did ours, a real diagnosis will make a positive difference in all of your lives—you know what you face. I recommend these tips:

1. Listen to others when they say something seems wrong with your loved one.

2. Trust yourself if you think something seems wrong with your loved one.

3. Write symptoms down so you can share them with a doctor.

4. Press the doctors for the steps necessary to get to a real diagnosis and stay flexible.

5. Ask the doctor for their level of certainty.

6. If your loved one is resistant to an exam or the diagnosis, change your language toward the symptoms, not the person. Know the dementia may make them unable to reason it or see it, or they know it but are scared to admit it. Show love.

Maureen was quiet those next few days. I did not bring the issue up with her. I wanted to give her time to process it. I simply implemented workarounds for anything that gave her trouble. I showered her with affection and did not bring up her struggles.

She broached the subject first. "Am I getting stupid?"

"No baby. You are smart. You will always be smart. You are just having a harder time telling yourself to do things. You know in your head what you want to do, but you just have a hard time telling your hands and your mouth," I tried to explain. I was reading a lot while alone. I wanted to understand FTD.

Her memory seemed fine. When prompted, she remembered dates, appointments, people's birthdays, etc., but she had a hard time sorting through her mind to pull that information forward. It LOOKED like she did not remember. I likened it in my mind to her file structure having a busted link with the data caught inside. When that happens, you have to implement a workaround to access the data. We started doing that together: we found workarounds.

At this time, her personality remained unchanged, save for becoming a bit quieter. She had a hard time with tasks that required multiple steps. She still drove initially, as over time that knowledge goes from the front of your brain (the sort of reasoning it out/problem-solving part), to the center of your brain where things become more instinctual. I would occasionally ride with her as a passenger to gauge when I thought she started making unsafe choices. She remained good for a year, but then we realized she could no longer judge when to make a turn well. At that time, we both agreed she should not drive anymore. Others might have fought to give up the keys. She did not. She said, "I don't want to hurt someone." That kind of selfless caring defined her demeanor, always.

She loved her coffee, but that became increasingly hard too.

We had moved to a K-cup style much earlier before the FTD came about. It takes far more steps than one realizes. Seeing her frozen in front of it, I walked her through the process and took pictures of her hand doing each step. I then printed them out and taped them to the counter with the numbers one through six.

That worked for a few weeks, but then no longer. She kept deteriorating. We got a regular coffee maker. I would put in the grounds and water and everything and have it ready for her to just turn on, with her cup and sugar nearby. That worked, until it didn't. I used a timer to have it run the coffee just before she normally got up. She would not understand that it had brewed in the kitchen, and I would find it all still in the carafe when I got home.

I bought a hot water maker and put it in our bedroom. She only needed to hit a switch, and it would heat the water. Her instant coffee, sugar, and a spoon would be ready in the cup. That too worked, but only for a while.

Lastly, I changed to making her coffee each morning and putting it in a thermos to keep it hot, so she just had to take off the cap and pour it into the prepared cup. Again, it worked, and then it did not.

Eventually, I just brought her Starbucks coffee or her chai teas during the week, whenever I could take a break from work. For sixteen years, I had made her coffee or took her out to her beloved Starbucks on the weekends. I made sure to keep doing that every weekend—on that point, we never skipped a step.

Our whole marriage, I would order our drinks and pastries. Sometimes she would stand in line with me, or, on crowded days, we would find a table together, and I would confirm her order, get in line, place the order, come back to the table for a kiss until they called our name, then grab the drinks and pastries and bring them to her. I always did this. Never out of control or a lack of trust—just because she deserved to feel special and cherished, even in the simplest of tasks.

Maureen and I had been planning to drive Route 66 in September that year. I asked her if we should still do that. She still remained highly functional in many ways, and said yes, she would like that. We made it happen. We took a month together, just us, in a really nice rental car and no schedule. We could take as long or as short as she wanted each day.

While she enjoyed the trip immensely, she did get disoriented by sleeping in a new place each night. I found I needed to handle ALL the details, which worked fine. Our marriage had teed that up well, so we just lived it. Early on, I forgot to check if she had her favorite watch on. She had only had it six months, so she got it around the time the symptoms started. It had a big face that she really liked (she said the style today meant "big-faced watches"). As such, we had to double back a hundred miles. I made sure to take that on as my bad to keep her from getting down on herself or overly worrying about the FTD. Each morning since, I would add that to my checklist.

The trip included many firsts for Maureen, and she could still take in each experience. It really came down to emotions and wants for her. We did not read on the history of things, as that no longer held any relevance for her. It became just a sensory trip for her:

seeing, touching, tasting, hearing. We had the Beach Boys, Elvis, or the Beatles going most of the trip, throwing in a little Huey Lewis or Cyndi Lauper for fun.

We drove from Portland, Oregon to Chicago, catching Yellowstone, Mount Rushmore, Devils' Tower, Sturgis, and more along the way. From Chicago, we drove every inch of Route 66 to Santa Monica—catching all the little towns, car museums, historic motels, and places of interest on the way.

As the trip rolled on, I found it was less successful for me to ask her if she wanted to stop somewhere than to actually just stop and then gauge her interest to know when to leave. She just had no ability to understand my question, "Do you want to stop in the Lincoln Museum?" I would watch her smiles and her mood and adjust accordingly. She was still a delight throughout the trip. However, I needed to think about food and drink and restrooms frequently, as the process of when and where had by then gone beyond her mindset.

We stayed in some of the classic motels, like The Blue Swallow and the Wigwam. She gave me the funniest look when we pulled up to the teepees at the Wigwam, "We are staying here??" We also stopped at the New Mexico State Fair. She did not process the meaning of these things, she just knew whether she enjoyed them or not. We danced to some music at the fair. If the FTD weighed on her mind, she did not show it that night. She just smiled and danced with me.

We stopped at the Grand Canyon on the way, and she wanted to walk down. My habit of never telling my wife no had to get adjusted. I suggested we walk down just a short distance. As neither of us had kept in shape, I did not want us to go down further than we could make it back up. I had to put the brakes on when I thought we had gone far enough. She agreed eventually, but I had left it a little too long. It proved quite the hike back up, with lots of stops along the way. She got agitated and tired from the heat and was unable to reason the dilemma. With encouragement, we forged ahead and eventually made it back to the top. I could see then that I needed to be more of a guide than a pleaser. Our relationship would have to change slightly.

Once at Santa Monica, we took Big Sur up the coast and to the Redwoods and back to Oregon and home. She enjoyed it, and we accomplished the trip with few difficulties. People would ask about our time away. If they asked her what she did, she had great difficulty responding. If they asked her if she liked the Grand Canyon, she would say, "Yeah. It was big." Maureen could no longer incorporate narratives as part of her day-to-day.

That became our routine with FTD. We changed how we travelled or functioned at home or went out. Yes, we now had a changed life, but life did not stop. We did not let it stop. Just because she had a fatal disease did not mean that her life had to stop. We decided to treat it that way.

Whatever happiness she had experienced in our first sixteen years of marriage, she wanted more. She just had no certainty of how to go about it. FTD had taken that. She tethered herself to me—that made me happy to become her anchor. We hit life straight on, as long as we could.

One of her dreams included active support of a political candidate that she believed in. She just wanted to do some small thing. In 2016, she had voiced her support for Hillary Clinton. Among these new changes, the campaign called us to door knock and remind folks to vote (I ran for Portland Mayor in 2012, so PACs had me on every email and mailing list). I took Maureen to the center, picked up the clipboard, flyers, and stickers, and made our way out to voters homes to remind them to turn in their ballots. Along the way, we picked up three ballots to drop off for people that could not get to a drop box. We even waited for someone to fill out their ballot right there. Maureen smiled at this and felt useful.

We went for a nice lunch afterwards. "That was good," she said.

"Do you want to do some more?" I asked.

"No. That was good though," she mused and looked away. Another item checked off her list on what we both knew would include an ever-quickening clock. We had no idea, though, how little time we had.

By the Christmas season, Maureen was really struggling with conversations with most people but me. I explained to her mother that Maureen had some ongoing difficulties and that we continued to work through them. Maureen had always maintained a high level of privacy and did not want to tell anybody yet. She did not want people to treat her differently. She made me promise.

However, her mother tended to fill in the gaps through guesswork when she did not receive the information directly. She proceeded to tell much of the family that Maureen had Alzheimer's and did not have long to live. I started receiving calls about this rumor.

I sat with Maureen and explained what had occurred.

"Why would mom say that?" she half cried.

"Honey. It is because you do have dementia, and it is hard to hide that when you have coffee with her each week. You know your mother. If she does not have all the information, she just creates her own story. Understand though, she cares about you. She did not say these things to hurt you. She just jumps to conclusions when you don't tell her stuff."

Maureen cried. She had somehow thought that we could just keep it from other people. It embarrassed her. I knew eventually we would need to tell people but had not counted on having to do damage control too. We had waited too long. I had waited too long.

With Maureen's permission, I countered the misinformation with our Christmas letter. I explained that she had FTD and explained what that meant. I urged people to treat her no differently, to respect her, but also to understand Maureen would take more time now to process things and answer questions. I asked for patience. Of course, ahead of time, I reached out one-on-one to her kids, her mother, and her closest friends and family with more detailed information. Oddly, most did not want to know more. I felt the distancing start: good people not knowing how to behave.

Shortly after the diagnosis, Maureen and I sat down and created a travel list. We had not done that before but rather decided on destinations spontaneously. We had no idea what to expect and how long we could keep travelling. I thought this was the time to fit in where she still wanted to go. We created a five-year list of locations. Little did we realize that she only had another year of travel left in her.

One of the places on her list included Disneyland at Christmas. She had an amazing time. In hindsight, had we known the future, we would have gone to the kids for Christmas, so she could enjoy that time with them. For all we knew, she had several years ahead of her. She truly loved Christmas, and we should have made the most of it that year. FTD does not let you have do-overs.

Shortly after the first year, her piano teacher had to end lessons. Her personal situation had changed, making it near impossible for her to travel to the house. She had provided lessons to people before with cognitive issues, so I had to believe the truth of what she told us and not that she simply decided to pull away. Regardless, it felt like that with more and more people.

Maureen and I still danced many weekends. She had more difficulty with the steps, so we simplified them to the point where we really did not care about right or wrong. I only cared that she kept listening to music, dancing how she thought she should, and having joy. We danced. We kept dancing. I think we danced around the pressing truth that she continued to get worse at an alarming rate.

We went to Barbados (on her list) in February of 2017. She was still very functional but needed to be led everywhere. Maureen rarely started conversations anymore. Instead, I would initiate words to engage her feelings. I would say things like, "The ocean water feels warm. Do you like the water?"

"Yeah, warm. I do like it," she would reply. She had started to use my words in her responses as it became increasingly difficult for her to create words herself.

She had less and less ability to process steps to do almost anything. She still ate ok and still bathed and used the bathroom with only modest help. Picking what to wear grew increasingly harder for her, so I would just lay things out on the bed for her each morning. She liked that and would smile and say, "Thank you." Small changes seemed to work. I thought, just do more for her. If this stays as bad as it gets, we can do this.

I had such a naïve mindset.

After Barbados, I found her self-awareness deteriorating even more.

At home, she would sit in the front room for hours, just staring. She would only get up if she felt the need for the bathroom or when I called her and asked her to eat or drink something. I would walk her through those steps on the phone 'till I was confident that she had something in her hand. I would sometimes come home though and find her clutching a spoon with no food in sight.

For her birthday, I got simple things that we could set by her chair. I got her a chargeable handwarmer that I would charge each night and leave by her chair each morning. I found her clutching it most days when I would get home, even though the charge had faded. I also got her a colored glass paperweight. She liked to pick it up, put it in her purse, and then pull it out and put it back in again. She clutched that a lot too and liked to look at it and feel it. I placed other things in her purse and left it by her chair so she could go through things throughout the day and perhaps brush her hair. I got a small tabletop picture of a field of lavender and set it on the end table in an attempt to spur on her thoughts.

I would come home and find she had one sock on and one off, or both socks on the same foot. I would find her with her bra on the outside of her shirt. I would find she had problems in the bathroom and wasn't aware that it had gotten everywhere.

You do not blame them. You cannot blame them. The moment you lose your temper, you have lost everything. Those things truly did not matter in the greater scheme of things, but it pointed to her further deterioration. I had to ask myself, "How long 'till she isn't safe alone anymore?" I had to make some changes so I could care for her more. While our financials would not allow me to retire, my job sat at the top of that list.

I had the position of a principal at an international architectural and engineering design firm where I had worked for almost twenty-two years. I led the educational practice in my region. I planned, managed the design, and oversaw the construction of schools for the top school design firm in the world. We had over twelve hundred employees in multiple offices, and I spoke about school planning and security all over the country. Yeah, I had a great job.

My long hours and all that came with it obviously did not align with taking care of my beautiful wife as she started to decline. A year into her diagnosis, I could see that I needed to spend even more time taking care of her. I would try to shed some workload, but in that position, it just comes right back. I knew how to listen and problem solve, so I became the go-to guy to fix projects that went off the rails. Throughout our marriage though, we had managed those added hours. Maureen and I still travelled, danced, shopped, spent quiet moments—everything and anything together. If not working, I spent every moment with her—as I had promised.

However, with the FTD, I found I needed to shift my work-life balance even more in her direction to provide the increased care that she needed. I had no idea how to do that, until a random drive with a colleague provided an opportunity.

He and I had known each other for twenty years and drove together one morning to see a potential shared client. We talked about life freely, and I expressed my dilemma. He asked me if I would leave the role of a principal and the security of that large firm. I said I would, "if the conditions were right." He asked me what that would look like.

I wanted to go down to just forty hours per week (in lieu of the sixty) with half of those hours in-home. I wanted no more marketing conferences and no more than one evening meeting a month. I wanted no more travel and all my clients within an hour of home. I also wanted only two to three clients and not the dozen I had previously juggled. The hours also had to stay flexible for whatever needs arose.

He said, "I can make that happen."

I went to Maureen that night. While FTD had greatly impacted her decision-making and processing capabilities, she still retained the ability to listen to what I said and talk to me plainly about it. I shared the opportunity with her and explained that this had less certainty—less of a safety net. I would have to open my own business and contract with this guy—something I had never done. I told her that scared the hell out of me. However, I would create a home office and work from home a lot and increase our time together. I worried about this uncharted territory, but having done this type of work for twenty-nine years, I thought I could figure it out.

The details proved somewhat meaningless to Maureen (I tried to keep them simple). We sat on the couch together, holding hands. She looked at me and said, "You should do it. You would be good at it. I like you being here with me." She eased my heart, as she had always done.

I gave my notice.

Though my employer tried to talk me out of it and offered to make whatever changes deemed necessary, he and I both knew it would not last. The workload and responsibilities would slowly creep back in.

I chucked it all: twenty-two years and the security of a large firm and prestigious position. I went from a company of twelve hundred to a company of three—not three hundred, just three. In fact, since he just contracted with me, I really had just a company of one. I felt like I had jumped off a diving board into a very shallow pool. It petrified me.

I became an owner's rep helping school districts hire the designers and builders and overseeing all the details to make sure they got great schools. I had returned to the type of job I had started my career with—the same type of job I had when I first met Maureen. I find it funny how things circle back. It afforded me so much more time with my wife to care for her and enjoy her in the good times and the bad.

Do I resent or regret what I did? Not for a moment.

It worked. We got that valuable time together. I helped her more in the mornings when she needed the jumpstart. I flexed hours and worked from home a lot. We spent more quality time together. I found us managing everything better. I saw us beating this horrible disease together, until it changed again.

In October 2017, the next piece unraveled, and the behavioral crashes started. We had to teach ourselves a whole new dance.

Chapter 7

Anger And Joy

A s the doctor had told us, Maureen had Primary Progressive Aphasia, which effects the language side of things rather than the behavioral variant. This continued to ravage her ability to clearly communicate as well as her speech pattern and ability to use the right words. This reasoning function would also hamper her ability to figure out multi-step tasks or new things.

All my reading on FTD made me believe that it should not affect Maureen's behavior. She did not have that type of dementia. I read that occasionally, much later in the development of the FTD, some of the symptoms of the other variant might creep in. I thought we still had so much more time before that might happen. FTD made me wrong a lot.

In October of 2017, a bit over 18 months after we noticed her first symptoms, we took a trip back to Mexico—to Puerto Vallarta for two weeks. Normally, that time of year, the weather turned cool and pleasant, but a strong heat wave swept through the area that year.

On the first full day, in the early afternoon, Maureen looked at me and became angry and hostile. We were lounging by the pool.

"What are you doing?" she asked sternly.

"I'm just sitting in the chair here babe," I replied. "Can I get you something?"

"No, you cannot. I don't want it."

"Ok. Is something wrong?" I asked.

"I'm just going," she said with her voice rising. She stood up and started walking off, leaving everything except her towel behind.

"Honey. Honey. We can go, but I need to take these things with us," I implored.

"Why?" She turned back and said in an accusing tone, "What are you going to do with them? Where are you going?"

"Well honey. I'm going to go with you," I tried to reason, still not understanding this new territory.

"No. I don't know why you are here. I'm just going to leave."

I grabbed her by the hand to slow her departure while I grabbed sunglasses, bags, and more.

"Don't stop me!"

We were starting to draw attention from everyone. To others, I know it looked like fighting. I could tell in that moment that Maureen had started some kind of mental episode.

"Sweetheart. I just want to help you."

"Oh really?!" her voice was suddenly snarky. "Just how? You don't even know what you're doing or why you're here. I'm just leaving." She would say this several times and make to just go, but obviously completely unsure where to. She just started walking. I collected our things and walked briskly to keep up.

"Sweetheart. Do you want to go back to our room?"

"Maybe. I'm not telling you. You don't even know," she snapped, hardly looking in my direction. She continued her quick pace.

"Honey. The room is over THIS way," I tried to explain.

"Well just how do you know? Do you know where I'm going? Do you even care?"

This caught me so unaware. A cross word had never passed her lips before—I had never experienced this kind of attitude from her in our twenty years together, so I found myself completely unprepared. I had done nothing, but I also understood that FTD did not care. You cannot assume a cause and effect in the behavior. I had a hard time wrestling with that. I also had no idea how long this would last. I thought maybe the extreme heat had weakened her defenses and triggered this irritability. I needed to get her to the room. I knew I had a key, and she did not.

I stammered, "Of course I care. You're my wife. I'm your husband."

She studied me—eyes full of doubt. "I don't think you care."

"I do baby," I pleaded. "Perhaps we can go to the room for a while and rest."

"I don't need to rest. I need to just go. I need to go." She started looking around trying to orient herself in this foreign environment. She looked down at herself in her bathing suit and towel, "I need my clothes. I need to go."

"I can take you to them dear. They are up in the room," I negotiated.

"Fine. Where?"

I led her to the room. She would not hold my hand. She remained visibly agitated and always looking around, like someone trapped, looking for an exit. In the elevator, she began again, "I'm just going to leave."

"Well, let's get dressed and relax, and then we can figure out where to go," I said.

She breathed heavily, obviously frustrated with me, the situation, and everything. We got to the room, and I said, "Here we are." She pushed on the door before I had unlocked it. I got the key out of my pocket and opened the door. She barged in past me. "It's cold in here!" she yelled. They had the air conditioning running for quite some time due to the heat outside—an admittedly stark contrast in temperature. I suggested that we get some dry clothes on her.

"Where are they? In here I suppose. Where did you put them?"

I opened the suitcase and started to pull out some appropriate clothing. She pushed me aside and said nothing. I let her work through it.

I then saw the obsessive-compulsive part of the disease. She would take something out and unfold it, then fold it, then unfold it, then fold it, and so on. She would do that several times and then grab something else that was familiar and do it again. While upset and agitated, Maureen also seemed to keep working through it in her head. She wandered the room looking at random things in the room. The room decorations included a small vase with rocks in it. She scanned it and said, "That's stupid. I don't know why that's here."

I replied, "It's just a decoration that they put in the room sweetheart."

She looked up and around the room as if studying the worthiness of this resort suite. "It's just stupid. I'm just going to leave."

"Where will you go dear?" I asked. I knew full well of course that I would not let her go alone.

"You'll see," she said and went back to the clothes, which she continued to fold and unfold several times. This went on for several minutes, and I gave her some space. I watched though, intent on this new behavior. Eventually, she threw one of the articles down in a huff and turned back to me, "What are you doing?"

"I'm just sitting here dear. Can I get you something?" I asked.

"No." She started pacing. I brought some water to her. She took a drink, then set it back on the counter, all the time not wanting to make eye contact, or when she did, she glared at me. She had not changed out of her swimsuit, which was still damp, so she was cold for sure. I handed her a robe. "What's this?" She studied it, not really looking for an answer from me. She threw it down on a counter and went back to her suitcase of clothes, pulling items out and folding them and unfolding them and so on.

Now over an hour into the episode, she decided she had to go to the bathroom. I offered to lay out her clothes—more so, I just did it. I grabbed the ones she seemed to fixate on the most and put them on the bathroom counter. Then I gave her some space. She came out and saw them and put them on. She stood silent but moody and abrupt. I offered her a hairbrush. She gave the slightest "thank you" but remained visibly miffed.

She brushed her hair for a while and observed me out of the corner of her eye. She did not smile. She then made her way past the suitcase, doing some additional straightening of some kind, and headed for the front room. She stood staring out at the palm trees and ocean beyond. She remained silent. She sat down on the couch and brooded. She was definitely thinking about her situation. I could see it. She looked at me periodically. I brought her some more water and said, "Here sweetheart."

"So, what are we going to do?" she asked. Well, at least we had progressed to "we".

"Well, we could have an early dinner."

She said nothing. I sat there with my wife in uncharted territory. I had no idea whether this would end soon or continue, or whether it would flare up again at the wrong time. I offered to get room service to play it safe. I thought that if I kept things calm and kept her away from people she did not know, then we could weather this. I suggested some foods I knew she liked. I received a barely audible approval out of her. She kept staring out the window, thinking. Her mental gears were definitely turning.

I ordered two meals I thought she would like. Among all this, I smiled to myself. I treated our whole marriage that way. She would narrow her selection down to two things, but then often could not decide. As such, I would order both things. This could be entrees, coffee shop pastries, beers, whatever. I have never had much of a preference—food is food, drink is drink. I would have her taste both and keep the one she liked. I would take the other. I always valued the time with her far more than I cared what I ate. She knew that and would smile when I would bring over two new beers (both with her preferred less hoppy and lighter amber) and say, "Here, try both." She delighted in my efforts, and the appreciation of what I did made me want to do it all the more often. As such, in this hotel room in the middle of this episode, I found it funny how things change but remain the same.

After the order, I dared to walk toward her and take her hand. "The food will be here soon. I love you very much," I said as I kissed her hand.

She turned and, with all her angst suddenly dropping away, said, "I know". She put her arms around my neck and gave me a hug. I kissed her on the cheek and just sat there a bit. I found the moment odd but tender. It felt like she had forgiven me for something: what, I had no idea. Perhaps she had just found her way back and was relieved.

Only later did I understand that she had seen the whole episode unfolding but also had no ability to control it. She watched herself in this movie. The obsessive folding became one of her coping methods to find something that she COULD control.

I decided not to broach the episode with her. The food came. We shared it and ate together. Things seemed ok, but she went quiet. She let me give her kisses and rub her back, but I did so with a level of self-control and caution. I had no idea what had triggered the episode and did not want to repeat it.

After almost a week of these episodes in Puerto Vallarta and trying to find the possible causes, I cancelled the second week, and we went home early. Something there, perhaps even just the foreign environment, seemed to throw her off. She went through a couple of crashes a day. I knew I needed to get her home to a familiar place.

I had no idea that these episodes would be the norm for the next year.

Maureen began to periodically get these severe mood swings. I would say she went to her "dark place".

She would get really confused and knew something just did not feel right. She always looked around her for the answer though— never thinking (or perhaps knowing and not admitting) that it came from within her mind.

She had control issues where she would still fold and refold a jacket thirty times. She would start mumbling to herself. She would have an anger and contempt for everyone and everything, including me. She would remember me but not always that we had gotten married. She would ask me often, "Why are you here?"

I would respond, "Because I live here. We are married, and I love you."

She would fire back, "You're a liar. You're just cruel."

These episodes could go on for a few minutes or two to three hours. They did not occur constantly or with the regularity of FTD's behavioral variant. At home, they occurred two to three times per week.

I analyzed things as they happened when she crashed in Mexico and after we got home. I also took her back to the doctor to observe and discuss it. She repeatedly told me that she could do nothing except to prescribe medication to dampen Maureen's moods. I held off on that to see if we could work through it another way. The doctor seemed surprised at how far along the FTD had progressed. What we had experienced seemed more likely for a mid-late stage development (not that FTD has stages).

Her FTD should have remained the language variant. She had a semantic type, which meant she confused pronouns (he, she, me, I, they, we), and had a hard time using nouns in general (everything changed to a "thing").

With the added behavioral piece, I observed in my beautiful wife certain triggers that I then tried to avoid:

- Alcohol of any kind, in any amount—we cut it out shortly after we returned from Mexico.
- If she got too hot.
- If she got in bed past about 7:30 – 8:00.
- Doing too many errands in a day—her limit was about two.
- Walking or eating in an overly busy place combined with being confined—i.e. small restaurants at peak times.
- If I let myself get engaged with technology or some other task that she could not directly interact with.

Maureen had what I called "shifts" and "crashes". I could see a shift starting, so I tried to change the conditions gently but quickly to avert a crash. I tried to engage her immediately by getting her up and dancing, or turning on music, or eating or drinking, or looking at something familiar together. Really, I just tried to get her engaged to stop her mind from wandering.

Sometimes I reacted too late, and she crashed anyway. For whatever reason, sometimes her mind just shifted into a weakened state and her defenses would drop. My adjustments then simply did not help. These episodes mostly occurred just before we went to bed, but also at other random times.

I referred to the verbal barbs and insults that she would throw at me as "soft needles": they lightly stung but left no permanent damage because I knew they came from FTD. I often reminded myself to respond, not react. Eventually, that became second nature. I knew her loving nature: she had no needles.

Most of the time, her mood remained in check, but I became hyper-vigilant in assessing every word and action of hers so as to counteract an emotional crash. Most of the time, the same loving person shined through. We still had many good times, but the speed that it had progressed at still alarmed me. I knew I needed to adjust our lifestyle more.

With just the two of us now and down to two cats, I came to realize we now had too big of a house. The kids just did not visit anymore, so the extra rooms seemed pointless. As I looked around the house, I saw that we simply had way too much stuff. Every room had lovely furniture and art, and every closet and drawer was filled with things from twenty-one years of dating and marriage. I saw it overwhelming her senses. She would start fixating on any random thing and then get upset for reasons I could not understand. I figured we had to find a way to downsize. If this meant moving to someplace smaller, perhaps with built-in care staff, that could help. We had to do it soon, while she could still mentally receive strangers.

That seemed to reveal another driver for moving. Friends and family almost never came around anymore. People tend to distance themselves from those with dementia. Our culture allows that to become the norm. This made Maureen sad in ways she could not describe. She would ask me about certain people and would not understand why she had not seen them. I would phone friends and create outings and visits when I could. Admittedly, our home sat in a wooded area with not many neighbors. This isolated her. I thought on a campus, she and I could see and engage more people.

However, I wanted to make the most of the remaining time in our home. After all, Christmas season (her favorite) had arrived.

In November 2017, Maureen saw a beautiful home with wreaths in each window in her *Victorian Home* magazine. She thought that it would look so beautiful. I thought about how many Christmases we had had in this home and how many we might have left. With this potentially being our last one, I would make it special. With forty-two windows, we would need a lot of wreaths and red ribbon! We managed it, and the house looked very festive. She studied the wreaths and ribbons and smiled. She used the word "beautiful" many times.

We went to Dutcher's Farm and got her flocked tree. I noticed her stop to pet the horses in the stalls. She stood still, quiet and thoughtful. She kept in good spirits though and really took it all in. Did she see herself losing her grasp and try to take in every beautiful thing of the season one more time? I think so, but she kept smiling. We made the most of it.

We continued to go out dancing as much as the crashes allowed us to. We spontaneously danced in the kitchen or front room all the more. I made her giggle and smile. Eventually, the going out to dance did not work. They started too late in the evening—one of her triggers. Our dancing at home, though, remained welcome and was our go-to option.

Christmas concerts also became a bust. She would start humming along very loudly or suddenly get angry, and we'd have to leave. I looked for matinees, avoiding the late nights. That worked hit and miss, but the crowds still triggered some crashes. I made sure to play Christmas music a lot that season. I also took her to see light displays as soon as it turned to dusk to avoid a late-night crash.

On Christmas Day, we opened the few gifts I had gotten her. Simple things like new tops and things for her to look at, as she sat so much when I had to work out of the home. I got her a glass flower, a small table-top Monet picture, and a series of picture books of great art. Her reading had progressively deteriorated, but she still loved to look and study.

She isolated herself more and more. Friends simply did not come around much due to their own lives. Maureen could no longer drive to her weekly coffee with her mother. As such, her mother would drive. After a few weeks of this, her mother commented to me that she had called Maureen to come up the driveway for coffee. Maureen said she would, but then never walked up. Her mother would call again, and Maureen answered and said she would come up, but never did. Her mother gave up and drove off. The steep driveway proved an obstacle in itself, and her mother no longer trusted herself (with her ailing knee) to hold the brake well enough to make it up and down.

Maureen simply no longer understood how to follow all the steps to leave the house on her own to walk up the driveway. This problem with the house added to all the others and reinforced my case to sell.

I arranged with my job to dedicate Thursday mornings to taking Maureen either to her mother's for coffee or to meet at a coffee shop. We kept that going for over a year.

At the start of 2018, I had decided we needed to start making plans to move to somewhere much smaller. A one-story where we could add care staff as needed. I reviewed places online and then drove Maureen to each of them to determine which places she found to her liking.

We quickly found that senior centers would not work for her. We went into one, and I turned and asked, "Honey, what do you think of this one?" As you might picture, it had multiple stories in a single building with a great room off the entry—comfortable, but sterile. You had this feeling going in that the average age far exceeded Maureen's, now approaching sixty-eight.

She turned to me and said, "I would die here."

I did not need to hear any more; we turned and left. After more research, I found that searching for "retirement living" turned up more of the kinds of places that suited our tastes. They had a lower average age, more energy, more services, and were generally more youthful. I had no idea at the time that services exist to help you find the right living facilities. We walked through this uncharted territory together with nobody advising us. The medical staff at the hospital knew about our search but had no such recommendations. I had not yet discovered FTD organizations and the opportunities there. We muddled through it.

We finally stumbled across a retirement facility on our end of town that seemed vibrant and new—Cherrywood Village. Maureen liked that it felt bright and cheery and had a dining room that seemed more like a restaurant than a cafeteria. They kept the grounds maintained and attractive. Maureen became fascinated with the fountain. They had a variety of types of housing.

We made an appointment and toured the facility. I explained our situation, and we looked at a few different units. I thought their cottages might provide the easiest transition. They had 1200 square feet (as opposed to the monster 4200 square feet we now lived in). While a duplex, we would still have our own front door, back door, patio, small yard, and garage. It seemed like a less drastic transition for Maureen than to go into a high rise looking for the "random tenth door on the left."

Sadly, they had none of those units available, so we put ourselves on a waiting list. That would give us time to downsize our stuff.

Our downsizing included so many antiques. Nobody we knew wanted antiques. Selling them online came with shipping hassles, so I elected to use a nearby antique mall and get a booth out of which I would sell them for a few months. I simply delivered them, priced them, and then let the mall staff sell them.

I approached it in earnest, hoping we might get the call from Cherrywood Village at any time. We started the downsizing process in January 2018. I went through each room with Maureen as best she could. She would start to get agitated if I asked too many questions or if I started to move things around too much. As such, I would take breaks with her, even a drive out of the house and a familiar walk to recenter her.

Short walks along the Foster Floodplain Natural Area usually calmed Maureen. This area sat just a mile or so from our home. Volunteers had recently restored it to clean up the illegal dumping and bring back the animals and birds and improve the quality of the tributary. We would walk for an hour and just smile and hold hands. We could then return for a little more purging.

In her most lucid moments, I would ask if I could sell this or that. She understood that we were moving most of the time. I also promised not to get rid of anything that she wanted to keep. This proved hard, as she started to become reluctant to get rid of most things.

The antique mall proved a significant burden too, and the money we made each month barely covered the cost of the booth itself. I took solace in knowing that the antiques had at least avoided the landfill. However, as tired as I became, that proved little comfort. I could see myself getting stretched thin, and Maureen's continued crashes at night did not help.

Mid-March 2018 these crashes moved to the middle of the night. She would wake up around midnight or 1:00 a.m. and go into the same crash mode, and I often could not talk her down. She lost sleep, and I lost sleep—not good for either of us. I tried a sleep aid (generic brand, over the counter, non-addictive, and safe). I found something light that would just help her sleep through the night. We started those, and they made a positive difference. I would give one to her at about 7:00 p.m. to get her ready for bed on time and not crash.

Neither of us wanted the drugs, but she seemed to understand that it would help her sleep.

In that same time period, Maureen would sometimes talk about people she had seen in the house. She would talk about people she heard, and I eventually figured out it came from the radio I left on or the TV we watched the night before. The line got blurred for her somehow. Confused, not fearful, she asked if those people had left yet or were still there. She wanted to know when they would leave. I would just simply have to say that they had left. That would typically end it. I realized less unsupervised radio or TV would work better. I since found others with FTD that experienced the same symptom.

She also developed a clear nasal drip. I later read that those with FTD commonly wrestle with this and with telling their body what to do. I had handkerchiefs on the ready and often handed her one. I thought about her "like a log" comment regarding tissues years earlier and chuckled at how I had not even considered a standard tissue anymore.

By early May 2018 (roughly two years into the FTD), Maureen rarely changed clothes without my in-person assistance. When I went to work, if she wanted to stay in bed, I would lay clothes out for her before I left. She would put on a sweater over her pajama top but remain in her pajama bottoms. Often, she just remained in her pajamas all day. Sometimes she had two different slippers on when I got home.

The daily physical challenges for my beautiful wife became more and more daunting. Though I found myself exhausted, I coached myself to not show her my frustrations and to never criticize her. She remained the love of my life and well worth being weary for.

I helped her change into clothes most evenings just to take her out to one of the few restaurants she still enjoyed. We had a burger place she liked, so we kept it familiar. We did not try new places as she got way too agitated.

We enjoyed Chevy's Mexican Restaurant for our date night almost every Friday night for several years before and during the FTD. Sadly, when the one five minutes from our home closed down, the other three all sat roughly forty-five minutes away, or an hour in Friday evening traffic. Her head sank when we drove up to our old haunt and found it empty. They had given no warning, they were open one day and closed the next.

As such, I drove her an hour every Friday night to go out to Hillsboro and found our favorite bartender Rudy had transferred there after the closing. Maureen smiled to see him. She liked their Blue Agave margaritas on the rocks with salt on the rim and extra limes: one proved plenty for each of us. She also enjoyed their fajita salads, though she would change the meats up between the shrimp, chicken, steak, and often the pulled pork. They did not have the pulled pork option on the menu, but they did it anyway. We often ended our regular dates with a movie, dancing, or a long walk.

We did those Friday date nights as long as we could. We made the margaritas non-alcoholic but still blue. We changed to a quieter corner of the restaurant. Eventually though, noise and the length of the drive proved too difficult for her mind to navigate without a crash.

In respect to FTD's symptoms two years into this disease, Maureen could no longer shower without my in-person assistance. I needed to turn on the shower, encourage her to get fully undressed, and place her in the shower. She would stand in the shower on her own, but she spent a lot of time in there because she lost track of what she had already washed, and as such would wash a few times. She knew to use shampoo and soap, but unless I stood there and walked her through the steps, she would use both on her skin and none on her hair. I later moved to a combined bottle product that was both soap and shampoo—one fewer step.

I found joy in spending this intimate time with her. When I say intimate, I do not mean sexual; I mean personal. I cared for her in a way that kept us close—closer than anyone. Sex really no longer entered into the relationship after the emotional crashes started. It just did not seem right to me. If she could not always control her behavior, how could I think she could make those kinds of personal and intimate decisions?

We kept the romance alive, though. She still liked to have her hair brushed. She liked me to hold her, to hug her, to hold her hands, and to kiss. I had to pick my moments though and watch the signs for stress, or I could quickly turn a shift into a crash.

She also started getting minor twitches or spasms. Not at all like a seizure, these simple twitches came out of the blue throughout the day and just for an instant, but they were very noticeable. According to my research, they were "myoclonic" and not uncommon with neurological disorders. They did not seem debilitating to her, but a nuisance. She tried to describe them as, "I jumped." To turn the situation when they did bother her, I would simply say, "You have the jumpys today." She would smile and say, "Yeah. Jumpys."

She had favorite clothes. She typically liked wearing sweaters, as she got cold a lot (as she had for at least twenty years). When I knew it was going to turn warm, I talked her into a long-sleeved T-shirt to avoid overheating and a crash.

She usually wore two layers because she did not like to wear bras anymore. As such, she would wear an undershirt and then the top layer. In truth, she never liked bras. Years earlier, she had moved from fastened styles to pullover, like a sports bra. That would have worked, as she would now struggle to fasten one, but she also did not like tight things going over her head and catching on her hair.

Even pulling off sweaters could bother her at times, depending on her mood. Loose undershirts worked best.

She preferred button-front pajamas, which sometimes meant she did just one button, offset the buttons, or buttoned and then unbuttoned again. Sometimes she let me help, but I tried to let her do it herself. With pullovers, she would put both arms in, though often one through the neck hole. I would help her back out and try again. She would get to a point and kind of stop before putting the rest over her head. I would remind her, and she'd go "oh yeah".

If she started to shift at night, getting her to put on pajamas became terribly hard. That spring, we had a few nights when I just stopped negotiating and let her sleep in her T-shirt or pants when I could only get her to put on one half of her pajamas.

She had only three pairs of pants that she liked. None had zippers or buttons. Two had drawstrings to tie. She could still tie just fine. It looked very instinctual when I watched her—no struggling. However, she would see the hanging strings and liked to tie them again and again. Sometimes she would tie those drawstrings four to five times a day. I then had to untie multiple knots each evening for the next day.

She kept them loose so she could get her pants off and on to go to the bathroom. I think she forgot to untie them before slipping them down, and then, when she finished and slipped them back up, she would tie them again. I would find drawstrings on hooded jackets tied with multiple knots. This likely came from that compulsive control issue like when she folded and refolded an article of clothing multiple times.

She liked socks, but rarely wore them correctly without me there—not that it mattered to me. I loved her. Sometimes she had shoes and no socks, sometimes one sock, sometimes two socks that did not match. I found she would hesitate after putting on the first sock. I would prompt, "And now the second sock." I did the same thing with shoes—"Now the other shoe." FTD impacted her ability to follow steps, and I think she sort of just blanked on the next step, or in this case the next sock or shoe.

She did not do make-up anymore except occasionally lipstick, which appeared random, whether in pajamas or dressed. She only brushed her hair when prompted, but seemed to enjoy it when she did. She had beautiful long blond hair, so soft. Brushing her teeth worked off and on with the paste on the brush and off the brush multiple times. If I put the paste on the brush and handed it to her while turning on her water, she seemed to do just fine. She liked the water running while she brushed. It soothed her somehow. If I did not follow these steps each time, it just fell into a jumble for her. It worked best when we brushed together.

She sometimes carried one purse, sometimes two, and sometimes none. Random things would end up in the purse, or I would find it empty. She clutched her sunglasses a lot and sometimes wore them up on her head. She knew she had nice Maui Jims. It registered with her, and she got alarmed if you tried to take them. Sometimes I had to free her hand up to take a drink of water or food. It became a negotiation to free a single hand. The simple steps of putting something down to pick up something else are very challenging for a person with FTD. As part of that control issue, she got possessive with her things. I tried to acknowledge that. Often if she needed her hands for something else, I negotiated with her and asked her to set the glasses "right here" so she could keep an eye on them.

She liked her wristwatch a lot too. She struggled to put it on sometimes, as it had a two-step clasp. We got it before she had such struggles. She really liked it, so we kept it. I thought to change out the band to a stretch-over-the-wrist style but was afraid she might pinch herself. She liked me to put it on her when I helped her dress in the morning but seldom wore it otherwise because of the clasp. At night, I had to put mine on the dresser on a washcloth (I don't know where that came from: it just started to appear on the dresser), and then I could take hers off and put it right next to mine. She watched and studied me doing it to make sure it did not get too far away.

> I desperately loved Maureen and still do. This, I realize, can sound like a lot of complaints or clinical analysis, but I'm really just trying to provide useful mileposts to those experiencing similar challenges or symptoms with FTD, or really any dementia. She remained an amazingly kind woman and loved me very much. She could not help her shifts and crashes. Love demanded my acceptance and assistance through her struggles. I kept her always in my heart and actions as the love of my life. She just got lost periodically and needed a patient guide.

I tried to keep her engaged. We often picked up the mail together. When we came home in the car, I would stop to retrieve the mail from the box and hand it to her. I asked, "Honey can you bring this in for me?" However, I would wait to ask her that 'till we parked, otherwise she would try and get out in the street. This request made her grin. She understood; she had a task.

Wherever she set the mail down in the house, I would read it right there. This was critical for her emotional state. I did not correct her or say, "No, mail goes over here." I let her put it down wherever she thought to put it down. She set it somewhere different each time: sometimes she set in the bathroom, so I would read it there. I would read it to her, as she had stopped reading altogether. I would tell her about a bill or junk mail or "A magazine for you honey." She felt engaged and still a part of what was happening.

Phones became problematic. When I had to work, I used them as my lifeline to her. Sometimes I could not connect with her because she had forgotten to hang up the phone from my previous call. I resorted to talking through the security camera microphone and listening through the speaker. I had to toggle back and forth on my phone app. It worked in a pinch. She would walk over and look in the camera where my voice came from.

She simply did not carry her cell phone and did not understand how to operate it anymore even when I got her to carry it. A few months earlier we changed to a simple flip phone, but she lost the capacity to operate it by that spring. I added a landline, thinking that old habit would kick back in. It did for a while. However, like I said, she often forgot to hang it up. I would tell her goodbye and then ask her to hang up the phone and then listen for it.

"Alright baby. I love you. I will talk with you later. Hang up the phone now please." I would pause for a few moments. "Baby?"

"Yes," she would reply.

"Hi baby. It's Scott," I would answer.

"Hi," she said so nicely.

"Hi. I will call again later. Please hang up the phone now."

"Ok." Pause.

"Honey?"

"Yes. Hi," she would reply again.

"Hi. Please put the phone down on the white cradle so it hangs up."

"Ok." Pause.

"Go ahead and hang up baby."

"Yeah," she would say. I would then hear a sound as though she had just put it down on the table. After a bit of this, I would just tell her, "Ok Honey. I will be home as soon as I can." I would then just use the security camera 'till I could get home later and find the receiver on the table.

She also no longer understood how to dial the phone, which worried me should she need to dial 911. I hoped the new facility would come with an emergency button, but I lacked the confidence that she could reason even to push it.

The call from the retirement living campus could not have come soon enough. In mid-May 2018, they called. They had a duplex, or "cottage" as they called them, available. We went together and looked at the unit. I thought it was perfect: wood accents, soft neutral colors, a small two-bedroom with a private back deck and lots of windows for good daylight. It felt cozy. Maureen also liked it and seemed to understand and not object. We had eaten at their dining hall periodically so she could get used to the campus. We walked the grounds several times, and she again seemed to like the fountains. The cherry trees that lined the street were blossoming. I wanted this setting to feel as familiar as possible for her.

A move will always feel like a big change for someone grappling with processes and new things. I made it a slow introduction. They gave us a month to move in, which helped to continue to ease her in with familiarity, though I had every intention of making the actual move in one day. I thought dragging it on would cause her too much anxiety. I picked a day to do the move while her dear friend, Candy, could take her for the day for her hair and nails and lunch.

While the staff had known about Maureen's symptoms since that past January, they still showed alarm at how far her condition had progressed since then. We went over tracking fobs in case she wandered off. She did so only once at our current home, but was quickly seen and turned around by our neighbor. We discussed the in-home care options. They helped us in every way and supported this decision. Perhaps in hindsight, we should have stayed in our home or made the move much earlier in her dementia. It had taken hold of her so fast. I kept thinking that we had to get into a smaller home, easier to navigate, with fewer distractions and with help nearby.

I also needed to reduce our costs or standing debt, given the likely addition of in-home care in the near future. The challenge proved daunting with so many things to take care of, each of them confusing and agitating for my beloved wife. I tried to include her in all the decisions so she did not feel like I just took over. In hindsight, including her in those details may have caused her some anxiety.

The love of my life spent much of her early years having decisions taken away from her: what school she went to, where she lived, what she ate, where she travelled, etc. Others told her what to do, and that weighed heavily on her. Always gracious, she did her best for everyone else—often putting herself last.

Later in her life, when we got together, she shared those earlier disappointments with me. They had really taken a toll on her confidence.

I committed to our relationship to give her a voice and to build up that confidence.

Making choices, though, was not easy for her at first. She would freeze, unsure, when I asked her where she wanted to go on vacation, what restaurant she wanted to eat at, what movie she wanted to see, or any other number of things. When you spend your first forty-six years never asked those questions, you have a hard time making choices. With encouragement though, she got there and even enjoyed it.

Sadly, not long after she developed her confidence, this FTD struck. I had to change the choices that I gave her. I resisted that a lot. I had spent over twenty years cultivating her confidence by letting her make these choices, and now FTD was forcing that backwards.

I changed my language from "What do you want to do?" to giving her two choices. "Would you like to do this or that?", or even a single choice of "Would you like to do this?" With the latter, I could at least get a yes or no. Again, I struggled against taking that last choice away from her, as we had built our whole relationship on giving her choices. But I also recognized that the struggle in her mind to sort out those choices had started making her sad—she saw herself struggling—more of FTD's cruelty.

I found we could still overcome those struggles with love and tenderness.

"Would you like to walk with me?"

"Yeah!"

"Should we dance?"

"Yeah!"

"May I hold your hand?"

"Yeah!"

I found packing, though, a bit of a challenge to make romantic. Purging closets of twenty years of stuff created emotional struggles because she quickly got disengaged and had behavior spikes. I tried to give her something to do while I packed or purged. I had her look at a photo album, listen to music, or eat lunch. However, she would hear the noises and start to get agitated. This made these tasks take much longer than they should have. I would often stop and calm her down, start in again, stop again, etc. I tried taking her on drives midway. That sometimes helped. I took her to a park to take a walk. The small circle of friends and nearby family could not help. They had their lives and even with an afternoon out, I could not possibly get everything packed in that time—even with a dozen such outings.

While the activity of packing agitated her, she did understand it. She understood moving and understood why in her more lucid moments. She sometimes helped me go through her clothes or our dishes to reduce some of it and seemed to participate willingly and with understanding.

A decision I both relished and would now caution against included giving in to her request in the middle of this to go to Disneyland. We had planned it well before we got the call, but the trip itself occurred late May. It went better than I anticipated. I expected the worst, so I set my bar low.

Yes, she loved the ultimate family fun park, but could someone with FTD handle it? Yes, but you do need to take baby steps. Maureen turned sixty-eight just before this trip. She had taken her first trip to the magical kingdom at fifty-two. Since then, we had probably gone ten times. She loved it. "It's A Small World" and "Tiki Room" would ring in my ears for days later: what we do for love.

She had seen her Belle music box at home and said she missed Disneyland. With her two years into FTD and six months into some real emotional rollercoasters, I suggested some local trips, but she kept coming back to Disneyland. Alarms went off in my head, "Danger Will Robinson!" We did it anyway.

When planning a trip with a loved one with dementia, especially to a place like Disneyland, I would suggest early preparations and low expectations. Make it all about them with these tips:

1. Go to this link: https://disneyland.disney.go.com/ gu.../cognitive-disabilities/. I love that they have this, though wish it said "cognitive considerations"—baby steps.

2. Plan only six to seven rides each day (yes you heard me) and pick slow and predictable rides.

3. Stop and listen to street bands—Disneyland has music everywhere.

4. Go simple (least stuff to carry) but bathroom prepared (wipes if your loved one needs it).

5. Keep them hydrated and fed—use open air spaces and tables or benches that are out of the way.

6. Frequently use the quiet break areas at the link above.

7. Start late/lazy and finish early—respect their limitations and stay flexible.

8. Know their familiar favorites—my wife had to start her day with Starbucks (in both parks now). We did Small World and Tiki Room each day.

9. Always hold hands and go to the bathroom together in the family units. I had considered an electronic tracker in case she got lost but instead settled for name tags (both of us had name tags to spare her dignity). We got lucky. Doing it over, for safety, I would have used the tracker.

10. Think open fresh air (Mark Twain, The Columbia, Disney Railroad).

11. Bring the meds and keep them on their medication schedule.

12. Find a hotel very close by to walk to—again, open air, no cramped shuttles.

We had a wonderful time (not without some challenges), and Maureen smiled a lot. I by no means recommend ignoring your gut and going to Disneyland if your loved one simply cannot do it. Only you will know for sure. If you want to do something special for your loved one, prepare for the worst. You will avoid frustration and can treasure the special moments.

I had many people and caregivers tell me not to go to Disneyland. I felt guilty because she had not gone to too many places due to her condition. We had changed so much of our lifestyle to get her in bed earlier and to maintain a routine. I figured if she got some enjoyment out of it, regardless of the crashes that would occur, it was worthwhile. She did not seem to remember the crashes afterward.

In May of 2018, her early FTD vacation bucket list would have us in Southern France, Monaco, and through mainland Italy, with Machu Pichu, Galapagos, and Easter Island that fall. I cancelled all those plans after the crashes in Puerto Vallarta the previous fall. She simply could not take it. She did not seem to remember we had planned those trips, but still wanted to get out. I risked it.

We had three days in Disneyland. We flew in Friday afternoon and back out Monday afternoon. She had crashes Friday night and Saturday night in the hotel room, but otherwise just some minor shifts during the day and evening. The way we did it would have driven any child bonkers. Every day, we started around 8:00 a.m. and finished around 5:00 p.m. with dinner after. At 8:00 a.m., we would leave the hotel room and go to Starbucks. As such we did not get to any rides 'till about 9:15 and there was no running from ride to ride—not a trip young grandkids would have understood or enjoyed.

We did Small World and Tiki Room each of the three days. As noted, they were her favorites. She could hum along to the melody, which countered the small confines. We also did the Columbia and Mark Twain ships, Monorail, Disney Train, and Jungle Cruise. Again, open air, slow speeds, and predictable outcomes. We watched the Frozen musical. We listened to street music, ate small meals and snacks, and watched people. We took lots of breaks to rest.

We watched the Pixar parade. We danced on the side as they played music familiar to her. She giggled a lot. We kept the pace really slow and relaxed, but fun. We had overcast skies the whole time and mid-seventies—perfect weather for her to avoid getting too hot. Yes, we had some shifts that started up, and at those times we pulled out of line to sit on a bench or get a pretzel, or whatever. I would ask her about faster rides she had ridden many times before (Matterhorn, Splash Mountain, etc.), but she pushed back gently on those, "No, those are kind of fast." Even with the FTD, she knew her limits. Oddly though, she asked to do the teacups (another prior favorite of hers).

Again, we made Disney a success because I spent three days reading her language. By this time, she had few words or would string together a word salad. I had to interpret a lot from her posture, eyes, hand gestures, and general demeanor. I would say this: knowledge came from lessons learned, but honestly, her changes happened so fast that a lesson learned one week became irrelevant the next.

> *You have to devote yourself to your loved one. You have to go all in. You need to watch almost continuously, learn, adjust, and keep nimble. That approach and vigilance will give you a chance at helping them through FTD.*

We dance with FTD. I do not mean playful dancing, swaying back and forth to your favorite tunes. I mean a pressure cooker sort of dance, like a high-stakes game of musical chairs, but people keep pulling random chairs out from under you. With enough time and devotion, you start to develop a rhythm. However, that rhythm includes being prepared for change each day.

That change became our routine, and we got good at it.

Until, in the middle of our packing, less than three weeks before moving day, she collapsed in pain.

Chapter 8

Crashing In

Scott's Journal – 6/2/18

It has been a rough forty-eight hours for both of us. About 5:00 p.m. Thursday night, Maureen was complaining of a stomach ache. I suggested she sit down and drink some water. At 6:00 she said it was still there, so I had her lie down and gave her one of her nightly sleeping aids. At 6:45 the pain intensified. She rolled off the bed to the floor and started getting the chills and some nausea, so I took her to emergency, fearing an appendicitis based on where the pain was located—right lower abdomen. Four hours there with urine and blood tests and a CAT scan and finding a urinary tract infection (I found later common for women with dementia. I will have to help her better in the bathroom). They also found some other anomalies they had to investigate and would be in touch. They gave her a morphine IV and a chaser pill to dull the pain, and a prescription for a week's worth of antibiotics to clean out the urinary tract.

Friday she was still in a lot of pain, and I cancelled work meetings and stayed with her. Pain all day. Oddly, the pain takes all of her mental focus. There were no crashes and only slight shifts, but on the downside, there was also almost no function. She was even more confused with words, being able to hear me properly or even see things I was pointing at—not so much not being able to see, but not being able to see and recognize. Also eating almost nothing. I give her a piece of food and she just holds it and does not put it in her mouth. I gave her two of her soy chai tea lattes at different times, and she just holds them. This afternoon I had to fork feed her pieces of watermelon. The pain comes and goes, but when it is there, it is all-consuming for her mind. I think it is getting better today.

Back to Friday, I got two calls for follow up appointments—pulmonary (they saw something in the CAT scan) and surgical—they too saw something. We went in Friday afternoon for the latter. The CAT scan showed a couple dense masses around and above the abdomen that they do not know what they are. They want to do some tests and draw some samples after her urinary tract is better and having less pain. One looks like it is pressing on a main nerve for the right leg, which could explain her past leg pains. They think it is liquid storing in a place that it should not. They are not sure but are taking it to the tumor board this coming Tuesday and will call me Wednesday with any thoughts they have about next steps. He wanted

The next few days, her pain had mostly disappeared. She could get around much more easily. The antibiotics seemed to clear up the infection. However, the ordeal left her very weak. She also ate very little and lost track of eating: I would hand her food, and she would just stare off until I pressed her to take a bite. Her eating had already drastically declined, and she had lost a lot of weight before this. I knew she never ate much while I had to go to work. I reached out to friends to come sit with her and encourage her to eat, but few could make themselves available. It broke my heart.

Tuesday, June 5, 2018, when I simply had to leave for a few hours (no work—no pay—no home) she apparently stayed up in the bedroom that whole time. I tried calling several times and looked at the main room security camera and never saw her, but I also checked the security system and could see she had never opened the doors. That meant she did not leave nor did someone come in. I had gotten ahold of her early in the morning, but rather than hanging up the phone, she unplugged it (again, confused), so I could not call her in the bedroom. I got home about 3:15 and found her just shuffling around in the bedroom with the door closed and the blinds drawn. I held her for a long time. She just seemed lost.

I really tried to maximize working from home and minimizing meetings so as to stay with her. Sometimes they piled up, requiring half a day away. I tried placing snacks right by her chair—all ready to just pick up and eat—fruit, snack bars, water—easy to consume with minimal steps and not perishable, as it might sit all day. I investigated in-home care, but I knew I had to stretch our money, not knowing when it would turn critical and how much we would need.

In respect to eating in general, I would say that first thing in the morning, not so good. Mid to late morning better—especially when she stayed calm. She had taken to lunches better than in years past. Dinner only worked if I found something that she still really liked.

She liked watermelon a lot, so I cut that up into small bites, and she ate that well.

She liked things in small bite sizes. She simply could not use both a fork and knife at the same time anymore. She still liked a fork and tried to fork everything—even things most would normally pick up. That could relate to the fact that she never liked to get her hands messy or perhaps the proper eating etiquette grilled into her as a child.

I would get takeout and bring it home more than I should have, but I also knew she had some favorites, and she would eat them. She liked this barbeque place that she often asked me to stop by. I also made her salads, vegetables, and chicken, which she ate well. I would get her simple things to pick up like baby carrots, fig bars, grapes, and berries. She had also enjoyed applesauce.

This all sounds like a lot, but she would always just eat a few bites here and there—not enough to keep the weight on.

She also stopped doing anything active. I took her for nature walks near our house on an easy, paved path. She felt cold a lot (even on a warm day), so I made sure she always had a jacket. I tried to get her out and moving when she could, though she had become so unsure of her surroundings when we left the house. At home, I danced with her every day, as that normally brought a smile to her face.

I talked to her about all our past travels, and she smiled then too.

I thought that she might enjoy the Portland Rose Parade that weekend, and she wanted to go. Crowds in small places bothered her, but not crowds in open air as much. If we could find a less busy place, and she could sit with a drink and just watch and listen. It could work. After all, we could leave if she started to slide.

I asked her every day about her happiness, and she always told me, "Yeah. Happy." Her actions in that week seemed to say otherwise, but I could ask only so many times without it bringing her down. She mentioned not seeing any friends, so I called her best friend Candy and asked her to come have coffee with Maureen that Friday. She agreed, but things unraveled before then.

Scott's Journal – 6/7/18

We were together. I forget the rest (paraphrased from Whitman).

I welled up but kept it together as she needed me to.

We had a doctor's appointment this morning regarding the CAT scan last Thursday. There were a couple nodules at the bottom of the lung right next to the diaphragm. They could not get a good look at them, so they need a chest cavity CAT scan to better understand what is there (the CAT scan was of the abdomen and had just caught a piece of the lung). We did not leave there with a sense of dread yet as it seemed so minor. I think her name was Dr. Vanni.

This morning, thinking we would hear some bad news, I had sat her on the bed when she was at her most lucid and tried to assure her, but also talked of the possibilities. I reminded her of a prior conversation where she told me that she wanted an initial effort to save her life, but not to undergo an extensive, drawn out, or painful process. She did not want to be kept alive in a vegetative state or in a manner that kept her from enjoying a happy life. While FTD had its hold on her, she assured me with the words she knew how to use, that she still felt the same way. We held each other a long while. Dr. Vanni confirmed that in Oregon, these would all fall to my decision.

I was expecting the call from Dr. Moran this afternoon, the surgeon we met with Friday afternoon, who had concerns about things he had seen around her abdomen in the original CAT scan. He was meeting with the tumor board on Tuesday and wanted to show them and get some feedback.

He said with such a clinical analysis that it is likely (not certain) that Maureen has a cancer.

He thought it might be an appendix type cancer that sort of casts cancer cells against the wall of the stomach (on the outside) and creates these nodules that fill with liquid over time. No idea if this is for sure what it is and no idea whether malignant or benign. Next week, he wants to have a short procedure where he makes a small incision and sticks a camera in her stomach and also takes a biopsy sample. He will know better then what it is and how to proceed.

If it is the type he thinks, it is a slow growth, low-grade cancer, and chemo is actually not an effective treatment. He would recommend a surgery that goes in and removes the nodules and then applies a sort of chemo patch over the area. The first thirty days after the procedure they watch carefully to see if it works. It has a 60-70% success rate. They cannot do the surgery here. We would need to go to San Diego. I do not know the timing of this or anything. I think we still move in two weeks as planned and just work that out around this new thing. After the surgery, she will not want to take steps anyway—better to get to this new single-level home and have care available as we need it.

I love my Maureen very deeply.

I got the call on my drive home from work. I sat her down and told her as soon as I got home. Her only words of acknowledgement were "Oh dear". I assured her I would be with her each step of the way and that we needed to hold hope for the best. We held each other and kissed. Her dementia may be of some help to her because she I think cannot fully grasp the magnitude of the news. She understands but cannot express it and her mind does not let her analyze it, so it is just a bit of bad news sitting in the corner of her mind.

Cancer. Wow.

All that she had gone through for two years, and now to have cancer. The doctor wanted more tests before confirming the type but suspected mucinous appendiceal cancer. He had gone on to explain that this cancer spits tumors out of the appendix that hang off your body's lining and are filled with a dense liquid. Whether benign or malignant, they do not commonly mean a death sentence, and people can go on to live much longer. He did, however, express concerns about Maureen's frail nature and mental state and how that would impact the options. We would talk more later.

That same day, I of course called her daughter, son, and mother and shared what I could. I phoned from the next room and played music for Maureen. They gave me mixed reactions, but I had come not to expect any specific response. I tried to do the right thing with them—all I really could do. My attention remained on Maureen—the most amazing woman I had ever known. While I understood that FTD affected her ability to process things, all in all, she took it much better than I did.

Over the course of the next few days, nothing came easy. Her FTD kept her in a fog most of the time. She had fewer and fewer lucid moments, and I treasured those. I still chanced taking her to the Rose Parade to lift her spirits. I brought comfortable chairs with canopies over the tops due to the light drizzle. We had nearly perfect temperature for her. I kept her well protected. She genuinely enjoyed the marching bands, the floral floats, and the people watching. She always liked to sit on the fringe and people watch. About two thirds through the parade, she started to feel tired. I could tell. I asked her if she wanted to go early, and she said yes.

She got tired a lot. I thought it might mostly be mental fatigue, given how inactive she had become.

We never did understand how the cancer might have affected other aspects of her mental state. The doctors assured me it did not. However, her mental state continued to rapidly decline, and new language and behavioral issues started.

Pronouns that she had swapped periodically for the prior six months she now transposed almost all the time. She started whispering conversations to herself. She started to count steps up and down the stairs in whispers. She became restless and had trouble sitting and relaxing or laying down. This got her mind stewing and then made it hard to calm down. It built on itself.

Anyone that tries to convince you that FTD turns the brain off has not experienced it. Instead, her mind kept searching for answers. It raced. She worked so very hard to sort things out; to gain control of some aspect of her life. She knew.

I found I had to change my speech to help her better understand—to better sort things out.

I would say, "Here, this drink is for you."

She would reply, "Oh, for you? Ok you can have it."

She would take the "you" and hold on to it and reasoned "you from me" meant "you from her." She had trouble personalizing it. She referred to herself as "she" a lot but almost as though referring to another woman. The same with me and "he".

I asked her if she wanted any more of her drink or her plate and she said that I could have it if I wanted it. She said it in a manner as though she thought I wanted more to eat or drink and as such asked for it, as opposed to reflecting on how she felt—full, still hungry, etc.

I changed my approach and language to guide her rather than expecting her to reason. I would wait for the signs of her no longer wanting to eat and simply let her know that I would now clear the dishes. I would play music and watch her response. I would still ask her to dance by simply putting out my arm and saying, "Let's dance." She typically eagerly obliged, although our dancing was more of a measured swaying those days. It still made my heart melt.

I honestly did not think the pending move or the apartment/cottage bothered her. I think she genuinely liked it. I would take her by every couple of days before the move to make it feel familiar. When she wanted to leave the apartment each time, she would stop and say, "Oh that is really nice"—often pointing to the laundry room (go figure). They had multiple minor repairs going on and floors getting replaced, but none of that seemed to bother her—she took it in stride.

The move would happen June 22, 2018. Her best friend would take her for the day. Candy knew how to show incredible patience and remained supportive of Maureen. Friend and family availability remained a challenge. I would enlist her mother more, but when Maureen's behavior would go off, her mother simply could not cope well. She did not know what to do or would get into "control mode" and wanted to force things—"You WILL do this." That approach often set Maureen back more than it helped. I found with the coffee dates that I needed to stay with them the whole time to run interference. Not to criticize, but at eighty-eight and old school, she struggled to deal with the rapid ups and downs that FTD brought.

Before the move, Maureen received visits from both her kids on different weekends. She smiled to see them but struggled to engage. I tried to coach them. These genuinely good people simply did not have it in their nature to engage her in a meaningful way.

Her daughter kept aloof. She arrived to pick up some of our purged items to sell for a fundraiser. She often talked around Maureen rather than to her. Maureen could not follow most of the talk so remained quiet and non-responsive. Her daughter would then loudly and slowly repeat it as if "now she'll get it." We all have seen people do this when speaking a foreign language—louder and slower does not help. Maureen also could no longer understand complex subjects and issues. The value and meaning and joy came from just sitting with her.

Her son came the next weekend. While also a very caring person, he stayed every bit as unaware. I would watch. He just talked very rapidly as usual with a myriad of words in every sentence all running together as though she would understand everything. He looked at a vacation photo book and then his daughters joined him wedging between Maureen and her son. It got too busy, and Maureen started quietly talking to herself. She then stood and removed herself from the situation. They did not notice. Her son said later that she seemed to behave alright. He did not see it. He did not watch for it. I did. She had low energy, got highly confused, and failed to engage in anything he said because he did not direct it at her.

I did not get frustrated with them. They did not live with this every day. However, I would have thought they would notice the change in her even more and look to adapt.

She received hugs and got to see them all, but they left as they came—mostly unaffected. Maureen as well—her focus seemed distant 'till she saw my arm and held it with no words. After those visits, I understood more than ever that really just she and I would have to make this journey alone—together, but alone together.

That coming week just before the move (that I would have stopped if I thought we could, or it would make it better) her condition turned for the worse again. She started that Monday with flashes of heat and cold followed by the shakes. I rushed her to the hospital for blood tests only to discover low vitals and high white blood cells. They kept her overnight.

I cleared my Tuesday meetings. I stayed with her Tuesday morning. She ran a fever, white blood cells stayed high, and vitals fluctuated erratically. They wanted to keep her another night. I cancelled my meetings for the week.

The next day, they changed from the camera and biopsy procedure in her stomach to just drawing mucous out of an open polyp near her appendix and multiple biopsies. It was just a small needle hole but was still considered surgery. She stayed another night. Still with a low-grade fever, she remained in the hospital. My poor darling. While with her most of that next day, I slipped away shortly in the afternoon while she rested to sign paperwork and pay our fees for the new apartment.

Friday, I connected with a mover who had an opening June 22 to move us. I also had the carpet stretcher come to the old home. He came late, which impacted a bit of the planning. I saw Maureen in the morning and then let her sleep, as she had had a rough night. They said she could go home in the afternoon, so I took her home after getting her prescriptions. We stepped out of the hospital at about 4:15, so I took her straight home. She smiled when she walked back into our home after ninety-six hours in the hospital for what had started as the shakes.

That last day, they said early results of the biopsies confirmed that Maureen had mucinous appendiceal cancer. I told her mom, her kids, and my parents. My heart sank. The doctor said whether benign or malignant (not yet determined) the treatment remained the same—pull those polyps out, as they may press on organs. Plus, you do not want them breaking open and having the mucous run around in there. However, they did not seem urgent about it and said it could be done sometime in the next couple of months. We had a follow-up phone consult three weeks out.

I only vaguely understood that they still had reservations about any surgery at all, given her frail physical state and mental capacity. Perhaps they wanted to hold out for hope—or let me do so.

A hospital stay takes its toll on anyone, but with FTD, my beloved wife felt it even harder. It left her with tremendously low energy. She also now had problems determining whether she even needed to go to the bathroom. As such, I had her wearing absorptive underwear continuously.

I left her alone in the bedroom in the afternoon to sleep for a couple hours. I came back from the front room to check on her, and even though I had her wearing absorbent underwear, she had both peed and defecated in the bedroom. She had gotten up, confused, then balled up the underwear and left it on a chair in the bedroom. She had somehow put her pants back on backwards with feces on them. One sock was off and one on and there was feces on her socks and shoes as well as all over the toilet seat and bathroom. She never called out for help or said a word.

What do you do when your best laid plans turn upside down? You simply cope. I avoided any cross or corrective language: that would only have made her feel self-conscious and cause her to spiral even further. I got her undressed, hand-washed her in the shower, got her pajamas on her, sat her down in the front room with harp music that she liked, and kissed her forehead. I didn't say anything about the mess and kept her focused on the beautiful sounds. She deserved that.

I cleaned up everything and put another of what seemed endless loads in the wash. I had not had time to grocery shop, so I ordered a delivery of pulled pork and coleslaw from her favorite barbeque spot. I fed her, and we watched a little bit of a romantic movie. I took her to bed when she looked tired enough, leaving the dishes out for the morning. We lay in bed and she cuddled close to me. I played a couple of her favorite songs that had become ritual for her to fall asleep to. I stared at the ceiling thinking about this new reality we were living with. Oddly, I just accepted it—come what may.

The crashes continued—going on eight months since they started. The doctor had given me some of an anti-psychotic, Haldol, to take the edge off—only to use once a day or less. Neither of us was into a lot of drugs. We would struggle to justify taking a Tylenol. I used it sparingly, preferring the coping techniques that we had developed, and adjusted many times. I did not like to experiment with my wife, I preferred to address the symptoms and prevent them when I could. That seemed the right thing to do.

She had definitely dropped a notch in her self-sufficiency, and we had the move coming—a poor combination. We had to get out of that big house and into something easier. I just wish I had done it sooner. I told her we would look at getting in-home care once we moved and have it part-time to bridge some of her challenges. She seemed accepting.

As for me, I felt worn out. I slept and ate what I could, though I needed to sleep more and eat better. I failed the cardinal rule of caregiving—take care of yourself. So many caregivers that I know laugh at that. "When exactly?? How exactly??" Yes, good advice, just difficult at best.

If you find yourself in a caregiving role, I would offer that you try these self-care tips:

1. Simplify your life by dropping (or suspending) all discretionary activities, clubs, groups, etc. Your friends will understand, and you will feel less torn.

2. If you work long hours, have an honest conversation with your boss and see what can be done to delegate.

3. Use techniques to make the most of your sleep. You may only get a few hours each night—make them count.

4. Stock quick, healthy, and non-perishable foods for yourself. You do not realize how little time you will have.

5. Seek out others to assist to give you a mental break of being responsible for anyone. That pressure drains you more than you realize.

6. Write yourself notes to keep you focused on their care. I left our wedding album out—that was all the focus I needed.

If self-care really were six easy steps, there would be no need for the term. Life includes a myriad of nuances and challenges that fly in the face of self-care. I know. I hear you.

Facebook Entry – 6/21/18

Standing in our "Floating Gazebo" off our bedroom, I notice now it has a sort of church-like feel. Standing on that deck, your eyes are about thirty-seven feet above the ground. It is a part of many good memories. I should have taken more time to look over the trees at downtown and north Portland with a drink at dusk or coffee at dawn.

Today is June 21—the first day of summer, longest day of the year, and on the cusp between Gemini and Cancer if you follow that sort of thing. It is also my fifty-first birth-day. I meet it with a bittersweet feeling in my gut—not due to age (that's just a number) but because this is the last night we will sleep here in this house we designed, helped build, and moved into almost eleven years ago. Tomorrow the movers come and take our down-sized collection of life's artifacts to a retirement community with assisted living and memory-care opportunities for my wife.

I will be living with her and by her side as long as I can—'till the end hopefully, so I can take care of her through everything. You have known of the FTD the last two years. Well, last week was a hell week in the hospital with an added diagnosis for Maureen of mucinous appendiceal cancer. Google it for more detail, as I am recharging for the next chapter that has already started.

I love my wife dearly. This is simply another road where I hold her hand and help her walk it. I am no better husband (and hopefully no worse) than any man I know—I'm simply here in this time in sickness and in health, receiving and offering moments of love as they come. I never would have imagined the plot twists in this story. Best to you all as your summer officially starts.

I had an overwhelming number of things to do, and the house remained nowhere near ready to put on the market. I kept telling myself, "This will pass, and we will get through it. There will be some pain and angst. I just need to do what I can to make it smooth for her. If she is generally calm, it will go ok. I will cope with the added work."

I thought, "She has dementia. She likely has cancer. She has a tough road ahead of her. I need to always remain caring and supportive. I need to do what is necessary and not try to over-achieve—pace myself. I have no idea how long I have with her. I need to cherish our time. If I can make it so she is not in pain, not emotionally distraught, but comfortable even though confused, generally happy and unquestioningly loved, then I will have done my part in her ending days, and that is enough."

We moved on Friday, June 22, 2018. I could only make it a soft move, leaving some things back at the old house. I felt a little melancholy on Thursday, my birthday, purely for selfish reasons of not really being able to celebrate with her in any way. Maureen had progressed to a point though, and had for quite some time, where she had no ability to look at those dates with any understanding. I mentioned my birthday twice that day, and both times she said, "Really? Well good for you." She then went back to staring and processing.

I predicted that she would have a difficult time with the move given all the activity she would feel disengaged with. I knew it. Everyone around me knew it. I still thought it a necessary step to get her greater care and peace.

She actually took it ok, with Candy taking her for most of that Friday. As such Maureen did not have to witness the actual move. Familiar things would now simply reside in the new apartment. I thought I could manage those reactions with her. However, when I saw Candy and Maureen at about 2:30 when the movers had placed the last of the pieces, I could see Maureen had become agitated in the latter moments with her good friend. She came in a little argumentative, not the gentle person that she normally exhibited with Candy. The two of them had left at about 7:45 that morning and seemed in good spirits, but probably too much activity. Candy had always shown Maureen devoted attention and care but can also come off as high energy, which could, under these circumstances, agitate Maureen. She had gotten to a point in the FTD where she needed constancy and calm at all times. As such, I hardly thought about the timing of this move, but I also had the long-term good in mind.

Maureen worked her way around the new apartment—studying. She started with feelings and statements like, "This is your place. These are your things" initially but then seemed to settle in as she recognized furniture and objects she had picked out over the years.

Obviously, all the normal struggles remained. I still find it odd how quickly we get used to new things and accept them as normal. With all the increased medical issues the prior few weeks, I had hoped for a time where we could just go back to the dementia. The side effects of the hospital stay seemed to have subsided mostly. She occasionally got a pain in her stomach, but it stayed mild—requiring, per the doctor, only Tylenol. Again, I used the Haldol sparingly.

Her ability to comprehend verbal instructions continued to decline. She stopped associating words with activities—or very rarely did. The most common occurrence consisted of me asking her to please lie down and her saying ok and then doing absolutely nothing.

I then asked her again to please lay down. "Ok," she repeated. Still doing nothing, and, yes, I waited. I asked her a third time and tried to help her lie down. "Don't push me" or "Get off," she would shout. I wondered what the new neighbors thought. I then backed away, paused, and tried again. I tried to hit that bedtime sweet spot before a crash that I saw brewing below the surface.

She simply stalled after sitting on the bed and would go no further. I asked if she felt pain—no. It was like her mind could not comprehend a next step. I left her in the bedroom for a while so she could calm down and perhaps reset. I went to the front room and lay on the couch. She eventually (about two hours later) came out to the front room. I asked if she would like to go to bed now. She said yes, so I took her back to the bedroom again and asked her to lie down.

She again said, "Ok" and then again proceeded to do nothing. I could not, nor would I, force her to lie down. If you have ever tried to get someone to lie down, you will know what I mean—legs stiffen, they push back against you, and try to brace so as to NOT lie down. All the time, I had the understanding that she said she WANTED to go to bed. I did not want her to nod off while sitting, as I did not want her to tumble out of bed.

Eventually, I gained her trust. After getting her seated, I lifted her legs and merely supported her back – lifting, not pushing. I talked her through it with a calming voice and cradled her back so she did not worry about falling or flipping over. I avoided putting stress anywhere. While she resisted a little, it seemed more natural for her. That become an evening ritual after that—every night.

These processing breakdowns, as I called them, showed up for almost any activity and required constant persuasion with a calm and soothing voice. This included sitting, getting in the car, getting out of the car, eating, sitting on the toilet, showering, dressing, taking a walk, and far more. With FTD, it becomes increasingly harder to follow steps. She had a difficult time now with even a single step. She would hear "eat" and would think that she had started eating, but in reality, she had not taken a bite. I considered taking more than five to six bites a success. My poor wife.

I made the mistake of taking her back to the old house to pick up a few things. The absence of her furniture (even though she saw it every day at the apartment) threw her off. She kept walking the rooms, mumbling and trying to sort it out. I took her there because I felt like I had unceremoniously removed her from the old home. She did not get the chance to depart on her own terms. It unsettled her. Looking back, I see the fallacy of my thinking. I made the rest of the trips on my own.

That last week of June, she had a lot of struggles.

She only had moments of joy and smiles. I tried to maximize those for her, but she just found it hard to relate now. She struggled to take things in any sort of context. I blamed the new apartment, partly the hospital stays, and the new medical conditions going on inside her. She had a lot piled on her, yet she still tried to sort it out—to make sense of it.

Maureen remained strong inside. When you look hard at those with FTD and past the superficial challenges, you find this disease reveals the strength, not the weakness, of those who suffer from it.

She started to hang her head and slump as she walked. I tried to help her to stand up straight, but she just labored now. She started to make less eye contact. I asked myself, "Is she tired? Is this a natural progression of the FTD or something more?" I had no answers.

The struggle to follow steps kicked into overdrive now. Instinctual activities became obstacles. I would put toothpaste on her brush and turn on the water for her, then ask her to brush her teeth. She would seem lost, so I'd put the brush in her hand. She still seemed lost. I asked her to put it in her mouth—sometimes she would get it and sometimes she wouldn't. We worked at it daily.

Sometimes she wanted me to feed her and sometimes not. She would not think to eat on her own. I had to prompt her to eat every time. She wanted me to feed her but then had trouble telling herself to open her mouth. When I tried to help, she clamped down.

Going to the bathroom became a major hurdle. She sometimes knew she had to go, so would drop her pants, but her brain was not telling her to sit down. I would stand next to her, lock our arms together, and count down, "We are going to sit together now, one, two, and…" Sometimes we succeeded, but many times not. Other times, she would sit right down. I understood that sometimes the synapses would fire and sometimes not. Sometimes she would receive and understand direction or assistance and sometimes not. My frustration was with strategies that would work, then not work—never with her.

She once ripped my shirt in a public restroom when I tried to get her to sit on the toilet. I think it scared her, like she might fall, so she grabbed at my shirt to brace herself. I had the small of her back to guide her, but sometimes I think the problem-solving part of her brain started working in overdrive. It prevented her from seeing the easy answer. We all get that way sometimes—too close to the problem.

The cancer took its toll too. She had pain three to four days per week, and I gave her either Tylenol or the stronger stuff. It seemed to help. What about when I had to work? I filled out the paperwork for in-home care—but how long could we afford that with the house not yet sold? It took me 'till early August to get the house on the market (even with paid assistance) due to repairs, cleaning, and removing remaining items. Two good friends, Charles and Cam, made a large dent in the "purge" by removing things for props for a local theater, things for friends in need, and things for themselves. I had given them carte blanche to have anything left in the garage. They helped us tremendously.

I felt like FTD sometimes put our lives on hold. The new apartment felt like some sort of weigh station. I went through the motions of stripping and remaking the bed every other day when she wet it, washing the clothes, cooking the meals, or negotiating with her to eat five to six bites. I knew this was like what people with kids had to deal with, but kids eventually grow and learn to do more stuff on their own; they become more independent as time goes on. Sadly, my sweet wife did not. She instead lost abilities each week. From all that I had read, she continued to regress at a far faster rate than normal. With so little still understood about FTD, they admitted that they really could not define "normal". They could not identify stages.

Even my mother thought she understood. However, when my father got cancer, she could talk to him about it. Maureen hardly got the concept, so I could not share with the one person who I shared everything with.

My grandmother had some confusion and lapses in lucidity in her nineties. My mother went down to help a few times. No doubt she had difficulties and an emotionally trying time. However, I was watching the one person I held most dear in all the world slipping away day by day. As a man you want to fix it but know that you cannot.

I should not compare grief. Nobody should ever claim their grief as more profound than another's. It manifests individually for each person and really does not compare. Empathy in grief runs counter to such personal journeys. The best grief empathy I ever found meant just listening and staying present. Suggestions rarely helped. Our journeys have nuances that nobody else can understand.

My darling Maureen seemed sad, but she could not tell me what she wanted. Perhaps if she could, she knew I could not fix it anyway. I saw no obvious signs of suicidal depression, but I sensed she wanted more out of the life she now had before her, with no idea how to express that.

I kept trying things. Given the time of year, I took her to the Rose Gardens. She loved flowers. She expressed a little joy there, but just a smile, and she was otherwise generally not responsive. She seemed to become almost catatonic, despite me holding her hands, hugging her, dancing with her, and speaking softly to her. FTD kept her spark buried. It crushed my soul to watch.

Early July, Maureen collapsed. I took her to the hospital. The doctors found two things: the start of a second urinary tract infection and the fact that she was not eating enough. I needed to do better with helping her stay clean in the bathroom, but I also regularly combatted the "not eating enough" aspect. The doctor suggested introducing some less healthy but higher calorie stuff: cookies and milkshakes. He did not recommend these as a staple of her diet but said it would help offset the reduced quantity. He also suggested nutrient protein shakes, like Ensure. I would try anything.

Maureen accepted these changes (to some degree). We took the small wins and made them a part of her routine. Starting the in-home care would also help; having someone there to feed her when I had to work in the field.

These changes helped, but she had already dropped down to 114 pounds—a weight she had not seen for nearly twenty years. I tried implementing some of the recommended techniques to get her to eat better. It seemed to help if I ate the same thing with her. I even ate off the same plate. We finished a chef's salad together at the facility's dining hall. I learned to gauge when to put a fork in front of her mouth and when to pull it away. However, given how much she changed day to day and week to week, I also understood not to get too comfortable with any one technique.

Through her life, Maureen had always eaten better mid-morning to mid-afternoon. This proved the same for everything now—eating, using the restroom, taking a walk. As such, we leveraged this alert period in her day best we could.

Bedtime still remained an emotional struggle. I continued the same physical negotiations. I explained that it would help her sleep better. She would relax until the second part when I would say, "I am going to take your hand, extend your arm, and push your shoulder. I want you to lay your head on the pillow." Again, the locked body, the objection, and the pained look of, "How could you do this to me?" That look hurt me inside, but she relaxed once she lay down. Again, I assured her I was only helping. "This feels good right?"

"Right," she would say convincingly.

"It did not hurt did it?"

"No." Then the need to sleep would start to wash over her. We repeated this every night. I would get in the bed next to her and play a soft song, and she would move closer. Thankfully and lovingly, the same every night.

I would lie awake with one arm around her, staring at the ceiling. "Perhaps this will get worse," I thought. "Or perhaps it is just a phase. Perhaps this is the beginning of the end, and I will sadly have to place her in a home." I did not even know what that looked like or how it would affect her. I hoped that day would never come.

They say you shouldn't care-give when you get tired. You cannot give your best. True, but I also found that I was less frustrated when I was tired. I was so worn out that I no longer worried about the crises. One event or day simply blurred into the next.

One morning, I gave Maureen a shower to wash her hair (she would see her mom that day) and get the smell off her from soiling herself. I had her completely undressed in the bathroom and turned around to test the shower water temperature. I turned back, and she was standing right next to the toilet just urinating on the floor—completely oblivious to it. My tired reaction? I just let her finish. I made a comment about next time, let us try to sit on the toilet (more instructive than anything else). I asked her to step in the shower and then just got some towels and disinfectant and cleaned it up. I then returned to her to help her bathe, then dry, then dress, and I never raised my voice once during all of that. I found myself growing as a caregiver, or as I said, maybe I was just tired. Perhaps our love simply triumphed over the struggles. I do not know.

Sometimes she would fight things, as the behavioral episodes that started the prior fall still remained. Maureen had them less frequently now, though. She often clamped her mouth shut during meals, grabbed clothes I was trying to get off or on her, would not raise her feet to step out of or into pants, etc. It felt like a bit of stubbornness, but likely also a bit of fear and embarrassment. I had developed a whole new level of patience those last couple of years, and even another level in those recent weeks. Mostly, she stayed sweet, sensitive, and caring. She would hold my hand when I reached for hers or let me hold her close as we danced in the front room, making all the bad go away.

She still whispered to herself a bit each day. I noticed too that she started to sometimes rock back and forth, which I had seen in elderly people—though it was just starting for her.

We had to cut our walks shorter and shorter. She got tired now just walking across the street to the dining hall, but we did it anyway. It got very hot that summer too, so that impacted her.

Our standard insurance did not cover the in-home care and adult day service. If we had long-term care insurance, it would have been covered—a lesson learned. The provider at the facility made the services available, but approaching $3,000 a month for full-time. I would have had to dump the other house first before I considered that. Hopefully, it would sell fast and for an amount that let me put a little in the bank for her care. HOPEFULLY.

Sadly, my sweetheart ended up back in the hospital for four more days mid-July.

She was feeling a little dizzy and weaker than normal and would not respond to verbal instruction. She functioned in a kind of fog. She also had a little shaking going on. Her white blood cells had spiked. She also lost another five pounds and was now down to 109 pounds. They conducted more tests and expressed more concerns about the tumors. The FTD had also caused her to mentally choose to hold her urine. I explained to them that that this unfamiliar environment was spurring on that behavior. I finally pushed for her to go home that Saturday, but only because they had run out of reasons to keep her.

We found that the medical professionals, while good people, tended to follow one set of protocols and did not adjust well to someone with cognitive disabilities on top of other issues. We found that FTD education at the medical level was poor in general. Alzheimer's awareness seemed like their standard training.

On this visit, we first met with a palliative care team. I had no knowledge of these services 'till they introduced themselves. They offered to help us cope with the changes brought on by Maureen's medical situation and recovery needs. They wanted to make themselves available for the road ahead with the cancer treatment and also suggested we consider moving her to a care facility permanently, which I resisted.

We spoke to another doctor, who said that Maureen should have surgery to remove the tumors. They found six: three hung off the stomach lining, two off the bottom of a lung, and one sitting behind the appendix. None looked like they had progressed to the interior of those organs. The doctor still seemed less worried and urgent than I would have expected.

We all remained concerned that Maureen was still not eating much. They needed her stronger before the surgery. Taking her in several days ahead of time would help with that, as they could give her IVs and get her strength up. The doctor also wanted to speak to the neurologists about the impact of the anesthesia. The surgery could last for as long as ten hours. They questioned whether the anesthesia would cause further regression of her mental state to almost non-responsive or vegetative.

This all weighed heavily on me, but fortunately for the love of my life, she did not take in those details. I bore them alone. I just wanted her pain-free and to have a level of normality to the rest of her days.

On the way home from the hospital, she made a very lucid statement. "I'm tired of feeling sick."

"I know honey." I asked, "Is the sick in your tummy?"

"Yes."

"Do you hurt?"

"No." Well, at least that was a positive.

The adjustments that you make start to become their own routine.

One morning, Maureen dropped a full bottle of chocolate Ensure all over the floor, which splashed all over her, the cupboards, the fridge, the stove, me, etc.

She said, "THAT made a mess."

What do you do? You laugh. Yes, she had FTD, but she was still the love of my life. I valued the latter as far more important than the former.

I chuckled and agreed, then helped her to change. I asked her to stand in front of the mirror and I brushed her beautiful long hair. I kissed her and said, "I will be right back." I then proceeded to clean up said mess.

People with FTD will make messes—a lot of messes. I encourage everyone with an FTD-suffering loved one to accept that with laughter and make sure their dear one still feels loved.

As someone wise once said (I think Robert Eliot), "Don't sweat the small stuff. It's ALL small stuff."

While she could accomplish so few regular functions on her own at that point, the FTD kept us guessing. On the rare occasion, she would still surprise me. When everything in her mind aligned, she would use the toilet on her own, use the fork on her own, or just get in bed and lie down. While these moments were fleeting, they were victories to celebrate, nonetheless.

But sadly, that did not imply progress. In late July, she wandered off.

With Maureen always having lived an introverted life, for a while I was able to go to work and come back, and she would keep herself to home. But deep down I knew that we were living on borrowed time, and eventually that would change. It did. One day I went to work for just three hours, and when I got home, I saw that she was flushed, which I thought odd with the AC going. It had reached the nineties outside. I asked if she had gone outside. She said no. A minute later the phone rang: the facility director told me that she had wandered off earlier. Residents and or staff had seen her and brought her back home.

In a bit of a panic mode, I got very defensive, which I shouldn't have. I blurted out some sort of appreciation but fought back at the idea of a change. I had no idea how I would implement the change I knew had to happen. They reminded me that they rented us this unit as independent living, and that if she could not do independent living, we would have to change to an assisted living unit, get in-home care, or place her in memory care. They encouraged the memory care, but I resisted.

I made immediate arrangements for a combination of in-home care and friends to sit with her during moments I simply had to go to work. At the same time, I tried to shift meetings so as to be away as little as possible. Neither in-home care nor friends could react as nimbly as we needed.

In respect to her cancer, the doctors now suggested that they should not do the surgery. They worried about the amount of anesthesia leaving her in a vegetative state. More so, her physical ability to survive the surgery appeared compromised. They broke it to me that they felt certain she would die on the table. They offered us no options. In the end, they feared they could do nothing. We could only wait it out and address the symptoms as they materialized. I spared Maureen this news. She could not process it anyway.

I did share the news with her family but received mixed reactions. I left messages for her daughter, who rarely reconnected. Her son preferred texts. I called her mother frequently to keep her updated. I gave her simple status updates so misinformation would not get out there. Often, she wanted more details than I would share because the doctors had not yet confirmed. This frustrated her. Telling her unconfirmed details as "unconfirmed" still ran rampant in the family network. I would then have to undo the misinformation, and I just did not have it in me.

Piled on top of that, the realtor reminded me that Maureen had to sign the eventual sale agreement. I knew that I should have taken care of that much earlier with a Power of Attorney. I had simply put it on the back burner to focus on more pressing day-to-day issues. I naively thought we could do that later.

Maureen understood we had to sell the house. She agreed. However, she could not answer a series of complex questions anymore, nor could she even sign her name. I worked with her with a pen and paper, but to no avail. I had waited too long—my fault. We went to our bank, which had a notary. Desperate, we went to see what could be done. We met with a very understanding young man who could see and understand the situation.

He explained that I could read each of the prescribed questions to her, get a verbal yes from her, and then make the "X" myself rather than her initialing. We did that and developed a rhythm. His understanding made that much easier. When it came to an end signature, he could confirm her identity from all the documents we provided. He also understood that she could no longer make the same signature. He told us, "Look. As long as she gives a yes, you can help her. Whatever mark she makes; we'll call that good." I placed the pen in her hand and held her hand. Together we printed the name "Maureen". I praised her and gave her a hug. She smiled with a bit of pride I had not seen in a while. I handed the paper to him and he said, "Good job" and notarized it. There still remains good people in this world.

We celebrated the victory as a godsend. Life otherwise kept piling up around us with the cancer, ongoing treatments, in-home care, friends and family being generally unresponsive, full-time work, her wandering off and diminishing cognitive function, dwindling finances, the home not selling, and most importantly, not creating a better quality of life for my beloved wife. Life spiraled out of control.

I did not want to put her in memory care, though that seemed the solution that kept staring me in the face. I kept going back to, "…together 'till death do us part." I know I feared memory care as the last stop on life's journey. You place your loved one in a facility that you yourself do not get to live in—just them. They are cared for twenty-four seven but also cannot leave unescorted. Care professionals address all of your loved one's medical and comfort needs, though in my research I found that services differed vastly from place to place. I could still take her on outings as much as I wanted and could still personally care for her every moment that I was there. When I wasn't there, there would always be nurses and staff around to provide for her needs and to help when she wandered off.

I told myself these things, but they never eased my pain—ever. I would no longer be living with my wife. Visiting every day simply would not feel the same. I irrationally craved for us to disappear together to a tropical island, but I also knew that to be neither practical nor responsible. I had to make some big decisions, but it made me so incredibly sad.

I wish I knew how Maureen really felt inside her head and heart. Other than lovingly holding hands, she rarely expressed her feelings anymore. I would try to not just accept her answers of, "I'm ok." I think she said that as an automated reply. I implored God to answer me. "Is she scared? Is she frustrated? Does she understand fully, or just bits and pieces of everything going on? Does she feel

I am betraying her by talking about memory care? Does she even understand what that means?"

I had two doctors, the facility director, the in-home care coordinator, and a caregiver at the memory care facility each meet with us over a two-week period. Everyone came to the same conclusion: not only should she move to memory care, she should have gone there months prior.

I hung my head, defeated, and took her to Parkview Memory Care to just walk around and check it out. I remember the date well—July 28, 2018. We looked around together, holding hands. The warm and inviting décor softened the sterile environment. The residents had an average age of ten to fifteen years older than Maureen. Living on campus as we did, they placed her at the top of the waiting list. They had a unit available in two weeks. It had a private bathroom, which I insisted on, as I knew she would desperately want that.

They furnished the rooms minimally, allowing us some customizing to make it as homey as possible. At just four years old, I found the facility clean and modern with lots of good daylight everywhere. The people seemed very nice, and one husband that checked his wife in when we were there raved about it. They had one of the best staff to resident ratios that I found in my research. Still, with the lump in my throat, I knew that we had reached her final stop. I kissed Maureen's hand a lot as we walked, but she seemed to just take it in, making no comments.

I could visit her 24/7—no restrictions. I could take her out whenever I wanted for as long as I wanted. I could bring her any food. It seemed I could do everything I would do with her that I wanted to. Except I could no longer practically sleep next to her each night or react to a mood in the middle of the night and just hold her. I would not witness all her moments anymore. I felt my role in her life diminishing, and that broke my heart. But I knew they could keep her safe and care for her better than I could.

How did she feel about all this? Would I ever know? Would she eventually not know the difference between life here and life with me?

Scott's Journal – 7/28/18

My heart is breaking. For all that I am trying to do for Maureen, I think I am failing. I fear she will be going into memory care, and I will be separated from her. It may in the end be the best thing for her, but it still does not make it any easier. I am losing my cherished wife.

My discussions with the surgeon following that walk simply reconfirmed it all. They strongly encouraged no treatment at all. They felt it would kill her. However, I also did not want to have her organs start to fail one by one, placing her on a feeding tube and dialysis. If any part of her mind remained at that point, I knew she would hate that, and so would I. Many years prior, we discussed something like that, and she asked that I wouldn't go to extraordinary measures to keep her going; rather to let her go.

Not ready to lose her, I cried a lot. I felt her ripped from my arms, piece by piece.

I made the decision alone. She would move to the memory care facility on a Sunday, August 12th. I would move out of the cottage on August 18th (not even two months after we moved in) with all our remaining things in our old garage. I would sleep on the couch in the garage to keep the house clean 'till it sold. I still held out hope that it would sell quickly. Only four miles separated our old house from the memory care facility. I would see her multiple times every day.

I also knew she could not have surgery. She would die from it. If by miracle she did not, the amount of anesthesia required for a ten-hour surgery would leave her with no more cognitive function.

These thoughts felt as though they would kill me. Did it hurt her too? She never said.

Scott's Journal – 8/1/18 (Letter never delivered)

My Dearest Maureen,

I thought about how we danced for years. I also thought about how you had to do a different dance before we met. You danced around all the issues in your life—forced to. You were trained to dance your whole life for someone else. You danced for what someone else said or did or expected of you. I know you asked through your first fifty years, "When do I get to dance for myself?"

You danced around your pain and danced around your unrealized dreams—rarely toward them. Everything is about steps to a rhythm or a timing. When it is to music, the dance is beautiful. The music changes, and the dance changes. You can be by yourself, with one person, or with hundreds. It is a celebration.

In the other kind of dance, you move around a subject. You do it again and again. You avoid it—avoid everything. Bobbing and weaving, you dance to this side and that. There is no music and nothing to dance toward. You have to learn to dance because you are not allowed to hit life straight on.

You stopped that kind of awkward dancing when we finally got together and just danced to music. It was expression and celebration—us and our love.

With the FTD, you got sick, and we had to do that other kind of dancing. We had to dance around what we did not want to face: the sickness was going to take you. We had to dance around it and focus on our love and each other. It was a desperate dance.

As the FTD shakes your mind, I have to figure out a new dance with new steps to help you still be who you are. I keep the music going so you never forget your true dance. I try so hard to give you joy. Behind the scenes, I go to the bob and weave and the adjust and pivot just to avoid crying and showing you how devastated I am. I want to avoid showing that pain. I want you to have only joy.

Your devoted husband

One week before the move to memory care, I felt the angst but tried to keep talking calmly and reassuringly to Maureen. I did not feel any better about the upcoming move. I knew when I got physically spent that she would still get great care. I read all the stuff on the internet to not blame myself and that this natural transition for Maureen would serve her best. These symptoms signified her time for this final step—blah, blah, blah. I would still desperately miss my wife.

I worried and tried to make sure that she never felt alone or lonely—even for a moment. However, for all I knew, maybe she had times like that right now with me at work or when she stared off or roamed the apartment or talked to herself or fell asleep. I did not know.

The surgeon had made suggestions to treat the symptoms and delay the impacts of her tumors. Rather than a full-blown and lengthy surgery, he suggested they do a shorter, less invasive one where they drain the fluid from each of the tumors to reduce their size and make them less apt to impact her organs. It would be a day procedure that they could do locally.

We would talk again after her move and decide on the draining option, as that sounded promising. They did not offer a cure, just a treatment to treat one of the side effects. As a low-grade and low-growth type of cancer, they recommended this path.

Before the move, I took Maureen to her mother's apartment for their weekly coffee as I had done for over a year. Maureen paced nervously and remained restless. Her mother looked surprised. I explained that she does that all the time at home. Her mother would just say, "Uh huh" and keep talking about it as though Maureen would return to "normal". She also joked, "That is why she is so skinny." I guess her mother just coped that way.

WEARY

Love is not hard:
Love is natural.

Distractions pile upon us:
                                    Money
                                Sickness
                                    Pain
                                  Grind
                                Fatigue
                                  Worry
                          Helplessness

These are to be peeled away.
That peeling exhausts us.

Love is the ever-present layer beneath
And is always worth being weary for.

Scott's Journal – 8/7/18

I explained to Maureen's kids (relegated to a voicemail and text in their busy lives) that their mother was getting worse and that we were earnestly looking at memory care. I was prepping them for the inevitable, but still waiting 'till after the move to tell them it is done. The move needs to not be a circus (from everything I have read and know of my dearest). It should just be her and I and a quiet time. I want to make it as easy for her as possible. It will be hard enough.

She has blessed my life in so many ways, and I feel like I am failing her now. I hope and pray she does not feel the same.

They bumped her move to Monday, August 13th because the director would rather that she not move in on a weekend with reduced staff around. They would get the unit ready by the 9th, so I could bring and leave some of her things on one of our orientation trips. We would do a little at a time, so Maureen understood, and it felt familiar. Even though she said so very little about it each time we walked the halls, she knew.

I had read about things to bring there to make her more comfortable and things to do to ease the transition. I would get her nails done Saturday. She would like that. I pulled together more current photos to keep in her room and some travel photos to serve as conversation starters with staff and others. I also needed to figure out what sort of decoration to put outside her door—something bright and summery—maybe a Hawaii focus. She liked Hawaii.

I kept myself busy to bury the sorrow. It still hit me daily. Periodically, I retreated alone and cried quietly for a moment. I knew that I would have a hard and emotional evening on the 13th, but that did not prepare me for the surprise the morning of the 8th.

I had never felt so scared in my life. I went in that morning to wake Maureen so I could get her ready for the in-home caregiver's arrival to watch her as I went off to work. I turned on the light and saw that she was still lying down, apparently sleeping. She had had incontinence again, but no big deal. It had become almost every day now. She lay facing away from me.

I went to the other side of the bed and gently sat down next to her. To my surprise, she had her eyes open. She just stared.

"Honey, time to get up."

No response.

"Honey, time to get up."

Nothing, but her eyes were still open.

"Honey are you awake?"

Then her eyes went from open to wide open and she let out a high-pitched, shrill scream that will haunt me the rest of my days. It sounded so terrifying. She then went taut in her whole body. The scream changed to a moan. The whole time her eyes looked right through me. She never acknowledged me or her surroundings. Nothing. She clenched her teeth. Her moan turned to more of a gurgling. I immediately dialed 911 while calling to her, "Honey— talk to me!"

Her body relaxed, but the gurgling turned to something like a loud snore—her eyes still open. The snore got heavy and intense through her gritted teeth. They sent the ambulance. Her eyes remained open and kind of rolled back. Then they closed, but the heavy breathing or snoring still continued. She labored. I picked her head up, pleading for her to talk to me. Nothing. I saw a bit of blood coming out of her mouth: she had likely bitten her tongue or lip or both. All this in two minutes.

The ambulance drivers got a bit lost but then turned around. I ran between the front door to flag them down and back to her in the bedroom to help her somehow. I could do nothing.

They entered. She was still breathing hard but seemed like she was in a deep sleep. She would not wake up despite six or seven people now being in the room. They asked me questions about drugs, records, history, etc. They all called it a seizure at that point. We just somehow adopted that as the room diagnosis.

They hoisted her onto a stretcher and into the ambulance, still in her soiled pajamas. I grabbed some clean clothes and followed in our car. I somehow remembered to frantically call the in-home caregiver to waive her off. I called work to get out of my meetings for the day. I left messages with some and spoke to others directly. All I remember is a frantic jumble—I was worried and unsure about everything.

I saw them get her out of the ambulance at the hospital. I saw they had her awake, mildly responsive, and looking around. She saw me. She understandably looked very confused.

Six and a half hours later, and they had no idea what caused it. They ran plenty of tests, but nothing. They still called it a seizure but never with certainty. They found the starts of another UTI so prescribed meds for that. They prescribed nothing else. "Wait and see," they told me.

I wondered later if she had just had a tremendously intense and frightening nightmare with her eyes open but still asleep. I heard some people do that. She told me years earlier that her son on occasion fell asleep with his eyes open.

That scream haunted me for a long time.

My poor baby. I love you, but I'm helpless to make you better.

The next few days up to the move were uneventful. She got much better. In preparation, I filled out pages and pages of her personal history and every behavioral issue she had gone through and continued to go through now. I provided general information about FTD on the forms the care facility provided. I tried to get them to understand her particular issues. They assured me that each caregiver would read it. I found out much later that a couple staff may have read it all, and some glanced at it, but most never saw those write-ups. That, to this day, remains the sad reality of care.

Scott's Journal – 8/12/18

Tomorrow I take Maureen to check in at the memory care. Today, we moved in her things.

This is quite possibly the last night we get to sleep together. I think she knows.

As we lay quietly in bed, I played her two songs she likes to hear as she goes to sleep: Peter, Paul and Mary's "Wedding Song" and Enrique Iglesias's "Hero". She lay against me as they played, and I held her hand as her eyes got heavy.

Afterward, I leaned over and kissed her on the forehead and said, "Good night Dearest."

With her eyes still closed, she replied, "Good night baby." She added, "Thank you."

I asked, "Thank you for what?"

She said, "I don't know, just thank you."

I teared up and said, "We have had a wonderful life together."

She replied, "Yes we have." I let her drift off and watched her sleep for a while.

Yes, we have.

Chapter 9

Memory Care

We moved Maureen in on Monday, August 13, 2018 at about 11:00. I walked her around a bit. I took her to her room. I walked her around a bit more and fought back the tears. I stayed with her 'till about 12:30 and then left her with the staff for lunch. I kissed her and told her I had to go to work (I did not). I slipped out in a way that she did not watch me leave. I did not want to leave her with that image. This made me a mess, and I needed a distraction.

Though we had finally gotten the house on the market with all the repairs and cleaning done, we still had a large pile of crap in the old garage. I planned to move our things back in there that coming weekend 'till the house sold, and then to find a cheap apartment next door to her facility. As such, I needed to empty and clean the garage ahead of that. I spontaneously rented a U-Haul for a few hours and literally packed one ton into it and then out again at the dump. I spent my anger at our situation with a lot of sweat and grunts, though the sweat was mixed with an equal number of tears.

Alone in the truck cab, I wailed. Tears streaming down my face, I cursed God. I slammed my fists. I cursed myself and this feeling as a complete and utter failure to my wife.

I held off going back to Maureen that first day until after their dinner hour so she could start developing a routine. I stayed with her 'till she went to bed and closed her eyes, and yes, played her songs to her.

Tuesday morning, I stopped in a for a few minutes to see how her first night went. They had checked in on her all night. She had slept restlessly. She had wet the bed, so they started using chucks (small absorbent loose-laid blankets on top of the fitted sheet). She smiled at me and seemed ok with things emotionally. I could tell, though, that she kept trying to process the wheres and whys of this place. I had told her everything many times before the move. I did not want to keep her in the dark. She said a few times that she understood and that we made the right choice and took my hand. However, you never really know how much they truly take in, comprehend, and retain.

I worked and went to see her again that evening, this time for longer. I repeated this on Wednesday, a brief morning visit and a longer evening one—each time 'till she went to sleep.

Thursday, I took her out of the facility to meet her mom for coffee. It started out ok, but she soon started to get surly. I took her back, and things did not get better. I left her for a while and came back in the evening but left before putting her to sleep. I tried to get her in a routine with the staff putting her to bed and to trust them. However, I could not help myself and went back late just to check on her and maybe watch her sleep. They had not put her to bed. I saw her wandering the halls, so I walked with her and helped her to bed eventually.

The staff should have done that, but they said they couldn't force the residents to go to bed. I explained to them that they would have to adapt. Maureen would not understand that after "tired" comes "going to bed." She would not understand the steps. Despite the pages and pages of forms and descriptions and FTD information that I had provided, I could tell that I would need to educate them on FTD. So much of their training included only Alzheimer's, and most of the residents there, in fact, had Alzheimer's. The two have very little similarity. You cannot play tennis with a bowling ball. All dementias have their own set of symptoms.

Again, I kept Friday morning's visit brief, then on Friday night I took her out to her favorite burger restaurant. She enjoyed that. We went back to the facility, and she had a good night.

Saturday started out well with Starbucks and a trip to the Rose Gardens. Before the Rose Gardens, I took our two cats to the Pixie Project—a non-profit pet adoption place. I called all over, and only Pixie Project could take them. I chose to tell Maureen this place would give them a check-up. She never asked about them after that. They could not go back to the old house that I had just had professionally cleaned. I had to sell it and had no idea where I would end up.

The Rose Garden went well, though sometimes with a little agitation. She enjoyed the flowers. She got hungry and thirsty, so we stopped at the vendor for a hot dog and a soda. She ate that whole hot dog, which surprised me. Generally, her eating had gotten better, though sometimes she did not want to eat dinner at the time they served it. I would go around 6:00 to 6:30, and they would reheat her dinner. I could then get her to eat most of it.

Her kids arrived that day shortly after we returned from the gardens. I warned them against too big of a crowd and that it might get too much for Maureen. It did. She started out ok, but forty-five minutes in started to get very agitated and then got downright angry and mean. She cursed and told the family to leave. After about ninety minutes, I suggested everybody needed to go. She stayed mad, so I told her I would come back, kissed her, and led her away from the door toward staff so I could turn and leave.

I had an aversion to her watching me leave. I never got over that the whole time she lived there.

Late in the day, I went back with just her son and his wife. Maureen remained upset. They left, and I tried to talk Maureen down, but she remained wound up and mad. It was late and she was in her pajamas. I kissed her goodbye and said I would see her tomorrow. She had simply had too many stimuli for the day. It overwhelmed her.

Sunday morning, I took her Starbucks and caught her in a much better mood. I left to "work for the day," as I still had a lot to move out of the apartment. I went back around 5:45, and she had not eaten her dinner, so they warmed it and I sat with her as she ate it all. It tended to often be a casserole kind of thing.

I had put a few pictures of her outside her room in a little glass case with her name in big letters—easy to read. I found that simply did not help. She apparently had an episode earlier that day where she went into someone else's room and started to undress, likely confused, thinking she had gone into her own room. Staff quickly got it under control, took her to her room, and had changed her into her pajamas by the time I arrived. She would need to be led to her room each time.

I sat with her on a common-room couch for a long while and just cuddled. *The Sound of Music* came on and she started to hum, so I took her to the mini-theater and sat her in the front row, where we sat together and watched it for a while. I then kissed her and told her I would leave now and wanted her to sit there and listen to the music. She seemed fine.

That was how our best weeks went for those first couple of months. Highs and lows became commonplace but still unpredictable. She would not think to eat, paced a lot, was confused often, but safe. Staff also needed a lot of training to help her and not assume she would figure anything out.

They did not understand that they could not just sit her in front of a plate and leave. She would not magically eat. She would look at it, confused about the steps required for eating. She needed assistance and someone to sit with her. You had to walk her through the steps of identifying her fork, of picking it up, of stabbing food, of putting it in her mouth, of chewing, and of repeating those steps. They had to understand that the prompting would have to occur over the whole meal. Otherwise she would stop and get up and start pacing. They needed more education—not just at this facility, but in the industry as a whole.

As noted, we listed the house. We had a glorious house, and I thought it would sell quickly. I had repacked everything in the cottage on campus and moved it all back to the garage of the old house. I left it all packed save for a few clothes and toiletries in some open boxes next to the couch. I would sleep on the couch in the garage 'till the house sold. I would then move somewhere inexpensive next door to Parkview. Even so, the house sat only four miles from the care facility.

Finances got tough. I could not afford both her facility with care and the old house mortgage. These combined costs simply exceeded our income. Each month would be a little drain to our small savings. I thought, "This is short-term. The house will sell, and that will build back up our savings, and a cheap apartment will keep expenses inside our income." Despite almost two and a half years of this altered life and reading countless articles and journals, I remained so naïve about how bad it would get.

Most days, I just ran on fumes. I cried several times a day every day, sometimes excusing myself from a work meeting when I felt it come on.

I thank Maureen for that—to have given me someone so dear to cry for. I did not cry easily before, and I did not know why, so thank you.

She started adjusting at Parkview, though she still asked almost every day, "Are we going home now?" I told her that we lived there now, but it did not quite register yet. I had not told her that we really had no other home and that I was living in the garage of our old house while someone else lived in the apartment. I understood that two moves in two months confused her. How could it not?

I think she saw in my eyes how tired and weary I had become. She looked at me with understanding and care. I loved her so deeply. Love also made me fiercely protective.

In her second week, she started to push back at staff. I typically visited her two to three times per day. I noticed her agitation grow. Some nights, I would change her and put her to bed myself, but others, I left her early enough to let them put her to bed to gain that trust with the staff.

On one of my daily morning visits, she looked tired, and they told me she had not gone to bed all night. They repeated to me that they did not force residents to do things, even for their health. I could not believe that they let her pace all night. I asked them to try and persuade her to nap during the day to keep her rested.

I went on to work and then came back at 5:30 and found her at the dining table, practically asleep in the chair with her hair in her face. They said they had tried to get her to eat, but I saw no food in front of her. They said they finally gave up. I wasn't paying them to give up! They said she had kept pacing all day and would not lie down. They asked me if I wanted to help feed her. Nearly asleep at the table, I said she needed to get to bed first.

I stood her up, and she leaned heavily on me and sort of shuffled to her room. I held her up the whole time. I lay her down in her bed, and she went to sleep straight away. I removed her socks and shoes and found her feet had swollen to twice their normal size. I brought the staff in there and showed them—it was obvious to me that they had not noticed before. We elevated her feet, and I asked them to put her on a thirty-minute check throughout the night. I thought, "How can they miss these things?"

By the next morning, her feet had shrunk a little but not as much as I had hoped. I asked them to have the site nurse stop in when she arrived. They called me midday to let me know that the nurse thought Maureen should go in to see the doctor.

Her doctor did not have an opening that day, and neither did any other physician at the hospital. I could only get an appointment with a small, affiliated neighborhood clinic that could not do much. I took her there. They checked her vitals but did nothing and said she should probably get an EKG at the hospital, so we went back to emergency and did not leave there 'till 11:15 p.m. They did blood tests to check for infection and an ultrasound to check for blood clots. All came back negative. They could not find the cause and suggested that we elevate her feet, monitor her, and let them know if it got worse.

Sadly, some days our health care system can feel like it needs an overhaul.

We monitored her condition for nine days. It did not get worse and eventually got better with the addition of potassium and Lasix as prescribed by her doctor over the phone.

She kept pacing. Even with the swollen feet, she paced a lot. When agitated, this helped her. However, it also burned calories, more than she took in. I brought more Ensure, placed more high calorie snacks in a basket at her bedside, and sometimes brought her meals in lieu of the facility food. I sat with her as much as I could to get her to eat.

I walked with her when she got too agitated to sit and eat. I would carry snacks and drinks in one hand and hold her other hand. She still loved to hold hands. Up and down the halls we would go, me putting chicken nuggets in her other hand. Sometimes she would eat and sometimes not. I did not want her to choke by walking and eating, but I also did not want her to keep losing weight. The staff, despite assurances before Maureen moved in, simply did not have the time to help her eat every meal every day. Too many residents also had needs.

I called late one night to make sure they had gotten her to bed, but they told me she had refused and started verbally and physically fighting them. I dressed and drove over, where I got her into her pajamas and then into bed. I rubbed her legs and feet with lotion and played her some music 'till she drifted off.

Those struggles resulted in a sit-down with management, who had become concerned whether the facility could meet Maureen's unique needs. They wanted their staff safe from physical abuse. While I understood that portion of their concerns, I also did not sit still for it. I had to advocate for my dear wife. I reminded them that they interviewed her, and they told me she would fit there "perfectly" (their words). I told them they had not kept up their end of the bargain. Obviously, all care staff had not read the write-ups they asked me to provide. I explained that their staff had not gotten themselves up to speed on FTD but treated her like she had Alzheimer's, so they did not align their care with her needs.

We continued back and forth a bit, but I held my ground without pushing too hard—I did not want her to get kicked out, as sometimes happens. For the sake of her mental state, I did not want to move her a third time. Those moves would collectively become too much for her to handle. They agreed to get better versed on FTD and to read her write-ups and to keep her on more of a nighttime schedule. She fought the most when she got tired. I agreed that we would reassess after a month. I also agreed to a low dosage of a mood stabilizer.

I loved her and missed her and wished we still lived together. Living apart did not feel the way a marriage should. I kept visiting her every day as much as reasonable, but still forcing myself to stay away at certain times to allow her to gain that trust with the staff. We lived a weird balance.

My whole life felt like a weird balance—a half-life. I lived in my garage and slept on the couch with an empty home above me. I killed three field mice that had taken up residence in the garage. I did not enjoy that delightful surprise at all, standing in my underwear in a dark garage late at night full of boxes with a thousand hiding places. I hoped that I would find no more, but I did still leave some baited traps out. I kept no food in the garage so as to not attract them.

The realtor held four open houses in the first two weeks, with very few visitors. They said they found August was often slow and that September would bring in more buyers. They scheduled a realtor's open house to try and draw attention to the home.

With so much spent on repairs and sprucing the place up, our finances got even thinner. I would have to watch expenses for a while. If the house sold soon for what we asked, then I could manage. However, only just over a year into my own business, I still wrestled with understanding all the tax laws. I had a portion of my home office set up in the back of the garage just to function effectively.

There was also, of course, Maureen's cancer. During the first month in the care facility, doctor visits and diagnoses continued, but they put planning for any surgery on hold. With her frail condition and dementia, the doctors would not authorize the procedure. Maureen had a near zero chance of surviving the operation and anesthesia. They even told us that after review, the alternative to drain her tumors would not work after all. They determined the liquid was too thick to drain. I reached out to the lead, Doctor Da Graca, and asked what to try next. He said we had to simply wait.

This did not affect Maureen mentally as far as I could tell. However, it saddened me to see her wasting away, with nothing anyone could do. What would take her first, the cancer or the dementia? Would she forget to swallow or how to swallow and go into an aspirating pneumonia? I had read that most people with FTD met that tragic end. I did not want that for the love of my life.

This care facility that she found herself in now, with a combined thirty-five other residents in two wings, unsettled her. Living with other people in the building shook her mind. She would hear voices or a loud noise and get concerned, and she would freeze to listen for it again. I would reassure her and ask, "Did you hear the crash-bang?" She had used this term herself for many years with the grandkids.

She would turn to me, smile, and say, "Yeah, crash-bang."

I would say, "It's ok. It's all done." That would redirect her.

During her pacing, she would see things on the ground and point to them or try and pick them up—sometimes just reaching at patterns in the carpet. She noticed the door stops by each room and would go to grab them. I would redirect her and ask her to dance or point to something up and in front of her instead. Typically, I pointed to flowers outside. Her mind raced from one thing to the next. I tried to focus her on real objects but did not correct her about the things that she saw only in her mind. I did not want to upset her.

This whole episode in our then twenty-two years together just felt like a long pause for a life restart. It just kept looping and never settling in—routine and chaos intertwined. I used that description for me. However, I often pondered what it must have felt like for my sweetheart. Did she feel the chaos? Did she feel sadness or despair? What did she think about when she stared off into the distance? Did she work it like a long puzzle or sit there completely aware of everything that went on around her with no ability to change it? I myself just sort of plowed forward with levels of sadness and exhaustion, but I did my best to lift her spirits regardless.

I would have some minutes of pure joy with Maureen when I would come into the grand room and her eyes would just light up. She would say, "Good. She, she, I, I am just so glad to see you." She would stumble through the words faster than she could speak them and happily settle her arms around me, holding me close in her frail way. She would say she loved me so much. I of course would reciprocate. These moments both warmed my heart because of our closeness but also tore me up because I knew, translated, it meant, "Get me out of here."

She did keep trying to adapt, but she struggled. I wanted to carry her away to a place where she would never hurt and never want, but that place simply did not exist.

With her rapid mental decline, weight loss, and cancer, I had the additional morbid task of writing an obituary, collecting contacts and pictures...in case. I knew that I could not do her justice after she passed: her death would devastate me. I feared the kids would not do her justice in my mind. They remained stuck only on the mom that they remembered from their childhood and never really acknowledged the person unleashed and empowered in her later life. They had missed much of Maureen's passions, strengths, and how she defined herself.

Her children came to visit occasionally. Her daughter every other month, and her son once every four to six weeks. I observed the uneasiness of their visits. This often happens when people do not know what to say. They typically ignored advice that I gave them regarding how to engage, so the visits lacked what might have otherwise made for happier memories.

Maureen's kids and mother just did not hear or listen to the details. Maybe they just saw that I kept taking care of it, so they figured they could keep treating her as they always had. Perhaps they found that easiest or more comforting than to face the realities. Not providing the daily care, you can take that approach. Rather than not engaging them though, I wanted them to feel informed. Occasionally, I would simply write them letters to capture it all. This kept me from needing to repeat myself or forget what I told one and not yet the other.

Scott's Letter to Maureen's Mother and Kids - 10/14/18

I wanted to take the time to summarize Maureen's current condition so you know what she goes through. I see her twice a day, so I see a more gradual change which might catch you more by surprise.

As you know, she has now lived in memory care for two months. She still has a hard time adjusting some days. On occasion she understands where she is but not why she is there, and that makes her resistant, angry, confused, or sad, or a combination of these. However, those feeling also pass about as fast as they come on. I think in her most lucid moments, she gets where she is and why she is there, and we talk briefly together about it in basic terms. However, even in these moments she quickly goes back to pacing, confusion, rambling, and remains unable to function independently.

What she says is mostly random words tossed together. She rarely uses nouns and confuses her pronouns constantly. Most of the time she thinks she said something, and the best response is to agree. There are brief moments where she hears what she says, knows it is not right, but cannot come up with the words she really wants to say. That obviously frustrates her a lot. I try to change the subject.

Her confusion gets into a mild rage sometimes. This is most notable in the evenings when the staff tries to change her into her pajamas or put her to bed. She has slugged and scratched caregivers and a couple of times me. She is simply lashing out due to her fierce modesty and her significant confusion. The caregivers and I show a lot of patience and try to talk soothing words to her, and sometimes we just change one half and wait a bit to do the other half. Sometimes it is just a lot for her to take in, but sleep and hygiene are critical.

Mornings tend to be ok. She wakes up rested. They shower her two to three times a week, and she seems to do ok. This was not initially the case, but it has gotten better. I showered her for the last few months before coming here, and she was good except sometimes when washing her hair, so I had to guard her forehead even though her eyes were closed—similar to pulling a sweater over her head.

She never likes her underwear being changed, but she soils or wets herself a couple of times a day and wets her bed most nights. She has gotten better about using the toilet around the 3.00 to 4.00 timeframe. She tells me or the staff she has to go, we race her to a restroom, and she drops her pants and goes. This is great when this happens, though normally it does not. They have tried to get her to go to the bathroom on a regular schedule, but she resists and then fights, and you cannot force her to sit, nor can I. She remains strong.

Something common in mid- to late dementia is happening to Maureen with her senses. More accurately, how her brain interprets her senses. She no longer uses peripheral vision. If something is not right in front of her eyes, she does not see it and sometimes looks past it, but this is because she is solely focused and concentrating and trying to maintain. There is nothing wrong with her vision, she just is only using part of it now. Her hearing is fine, though she cannot repeat back what you said. That is the FTD. She jumbles the syllables or repeats something that rhymes with it. Tastes—things are too hot for her now, so everything is cooled down.

Smell has to be right under her nose. Things feel sticky when they are not, or at least she thinks they are sticky.

Generally, the care team is trying to figure out how to keep her mood stabilized and keep her eating and sleeping well. 90% of the residents there have Alzheimer's, as that is by far the more common. With Alzheimer's they often revert to a younger child self. They are unsure and confused but often will receive help—even wanting it. That is not to say Alzheimer's patients do not lash out, become irritable, or yell—they do, but it is less common and tends to be more in their lucid moments, not the norm. With your mother's FTD, she is not reverting, but frustrated by her lack of ability to follow steps she wants to follow, to say things she wants to say, and frustrated at the confusion she experiences most all the time. It is like she knows she should not be so confused but is bothered that she is. It is a subtle difference but adds to her frustration.

Last year, this irritability kicked in about October and slowed a bit by March. It has increased in severity the last two to three weeks (October again). This may be the shorter amount of daylight hours and sundowners syndrome. We are going to try a mood stabilizer (psychotropic) to try and take the edge off. She will feel better and will be more agreeable to letting people help her—we hope. If it has no effect, we will take her off it.

The swelling in her feet and legs has gone down considerably. Her primary care physician prescribed a short-term drug, and that seemed to work well. As of this moment, the only thing she is taking is the melatonin at night to help her get sleepy.

Generally, she is feeling healthy in that her hip does not hurt as much, nor do her feet. She complains sometimes about her stomach, but other days, there is no pain.

Her eating is sporadic, as it is hard to get her to sit still. We have gone to some mobile food that she can carry with her as opposed to just stuff on a plate. We also have her drinking Ensure to boost her calorie intake. She is at 102 pounds. When we married, she was 114. Her heaviest was about 128. She was about 120 early June.

I do check on her every single night about her eating and sleeping. My general schedule is I plan to have dinner with her four nights a week and I tuck her in five nights a week. The other nights I call, and some of those nights she will not eat or sleep, so I come over and assist staff. There are probably only two nights a week where I do not have to come in and support the staff. That feels like it is changing as staff continues to work out ways to support her. I had a meeting with the director last Friday and discussed all issues and how to make improvements in her care. I will watch to make sure they follow through.

As for Maureen's cancer, it is proving to be inoperable. It is a low grade, slow growth cancer, so that is good. However, her dementia and very slight build complicates the options. Normally with this type, they do a long operation and remove the tumors. The doctors say they have no confidence she will survive the operation in her condition or will be able to pull her mind out of the anesthesia if she does survive. It is a ten-hour surgery and twelve hours of anesthesia. Maureen is simply not strong enough or doesn't have the mind to deal with that. It would take a minimum of three weeks in the hospital to prep her and build up her body, and she would still have a high likelihood of dying on the table. If she were to survive, there is a high likelihood she would be non-verbal and non-responsive after she awoke from the anesthesia and potentially bed-bound the rest of her life.

Chemo typically has no effect on this type of cancer. If things get bad, they might try some targeted chemo blasts or a chemo pill, but that will make her really sick and hard for her to deal with that, or understand, or mentally rally from it. She would likely need to go on a feeding tube or IV, but with her dementia, she would pull those things out.

We tried to drain her tumors, but never got the needle in. She fought. It did not matter because an ultrasound found all the liquid was too thick to remove anyway. She flailed a lot during the attempted procedure. They would have to put her out to do it, which they might if they think it will do some good. When they did the ultrasound, they found the kidney and liver to be in good shape, and the tumors had not grown. The stomach has us worried because the tumors are intermingled with the stomach lining and will cause her some ongoing pain and impact her appetite. We will manage those symptoms and work around them best we can. They want to see her again in January.

As you can see, it is really hard with the added complications to find a clear path for treatment.

I am not trying to paint a doom and gloom picture, but more a real one. Believe me, nobody wants her well more than me. It has taken its toll on me, but that is obviously nothing compared to the toll on her. We still have daily positive moments, so I cherish those.

If I ever think her health is fading fast, I will phone you. Right now, it seems to be a very slow descent, very gradual that I almost do not see it day to day but do see it week to week. Sometimes it looks like she is rallying, but then some other thing crops up. Nothing feels imminent to any of the health professionals or me.

She is getting great care but would rather be somewhere else. However, when I take her out, she cannot wait to get back. She has a few care-givers that she likes, so that helps when she is having a bad day. She does get sad some days and blames herself. I try hard to build her up. I tell her she is special; she is good, she is smart. She has lived most of her life with varying degrees of criticism, so she has very low self-confidence. She does not have the mental capacity anymore to "self-rally", so she needs that positive reinforcement.

The house has not yet sold and has been on the market about sixty days. Average turnaround here has been eighty days. We will see. Right now, bills are exceeding income, but just by a little. Dumping the mortgage and me getting into a cheap apartment will get us to even. I am also investigating with a CPA the potential for writing off a portion of her care. None of the long-term memory care is covered by insurance. This is not to alarm you—I will do everything possible to make sure it does not affect her care but want you to know that this remains a challenge.

As always, if you have questions or concerns,
let me know.

Thanks,

Scott

I wrote about Maureen's agitation and about ways of talking to her in the hope they would take those ideas to heart and perhaps have better visits with Maureen. Not that she did not have any agitated moments with me—she did. However, I learned how to "talk her down" but never "talk down to her." I simply committed myself. When you commit to someone wholly, you give someone 100% of your attention. You do not talk around them. You do not talk about them to someone else. You show interest in everything they say, even when it devolves into an undiscernible word salad.

Yes, she would nervously pace, but I loved those times: walking together, holding hands, eating together, talking with each other, and simply spending time in each other's company. It required a changed perspective and an unconditional love for that person. You live with a level of intention. My phone never came out (each time I turned the ringer off in the lobby before I came in) except to play her music, and then I tried to have it cued up before entering. That way, I could just reach into my pocket and turn it on as we walked.

I made it like a bit of magic. She would look up and hear her songs then smile and hum and hold me closer. In that closeness, we found our dance.

I had a playlist of about twenty-five of her favorite songs—an eclectic mix. It included Springsteen and Elvis, Sonny and Cher, Croce and Dylan, Elton John, Cyndi Lauper, and Bryan Adams. It included gospel and Christmas. It included piano like Brickman and Michael Allen Harrison. It still does on my phone today. I often select my "Maureen" playlist.

She would sometimes sing a few words, not always intelligible but delightful. I swear sometimes she sang the notes in lieu of the words. She could still carry a tune. She would hum to certain songs. That became how I edited the playlist: I listened to what songs moved her.

While I have many fond memories of our early days together, I also treasure us holding hands walking up and down those halls with music coming from my pocket and her singing along or looking up at me and smiling for one song or another saying, "So wonderful; that's just, just, just wonderful." Often, we would stop at the end of the hall and slow dance to a song. She still held me gently and swayed back and forth.

"We like dancing," I would say.

"Yeah they really do," she would reply or just insert a "mm-hm" into her humming. As I noted, with the FTD, she rarely used nouns anymore unless just repeating one after me. She frequently confused pronouns as above with "they" instead of "we". Sometimes she just spoke word salad like, "He needs it to go that way."

To which I would respond, "That way, huh?"

She would smile and answer, "Yeah. Yeah. It's perfect."

Sometimes she spoke more cryptically, like, "There that they are. They just just just don't."

I would reply in the affirmative, "You're right, they don't."

I had no idea what she intended, but it did not matter. I would repeat her words back in agreement, and she would grin, and say, "Yeah."

She felt in those moments that she communicated. That relieved agitation, boosted confidence, and made her feel just a little normal.

She typically delighted in seeing me, though a couple of times not so much. She might already have a bad mood going, and I just happened to come along at the wrong time. Sometimes also if I stayed too long, she might develop a bad mood and then would later come out of it. I had to respect that she went through a lot of emotions in a single day. I think it stemmed from a general confusion and a "what am I supposed to be doing" sort of feeling. Actually, I could relate.

She still had brief lucid seconds a couple of times a week during which she understood almost everything. She would say, "I am afraid. I don't want to die." Those moments tore me apart, but thankfully for her they lasted only a few seconds, and she moved on to another issue or pacing.

She continued to ask me to take her home for the first few months. It hurt my heart a lot to not be able to tell her yes. On occasion, she asked if I would sleep with her tonight: that hurt too. I thought maybe I did need to sleep there once but then wondered whether that would set a bad precedent for her and keep her from adapting. I also did not know for sure how that would work with a twin bed. Perhaps I could bring a cot. I could not take her to the garage for the night to sleep on the couch with me. With the bathroom upstairs, general disorientation, and perhaps a worry that things in her memory had gone missing, that seemed like a worse idea. I had to give it more thought, but it seemed possible. I recognized the importance of routine for her, but also those things that boost her spirits.

Residents certainly started to recognize her as one of them but still viewed her as the new person, I think. She did not make new friends easily. She also did not understand them and why she was living with them. She had a hard time relating just yet. One lady spent a couple of days holding Maureen's hand, which seemed nice, but then she started to force Maureen to go and do things she wanted to do—kind of like a bully. I kept an eye on her and told staff to watch them. I did not want to squelch a friendship, but I also knew Maureen lacked the confidence or the toughness to tell someone, "No. I do not want to do that." It eventually stopped on its own.

I also found it important to label clothes in the care facility, otherwise they would end up disappearing.

Did you ever go to camp as a kid and your mother would write your name on everything in a vain attempt to keep you from losing your stuff? You lost it anyway didn't you? I would end up coming home from those childhood camps missing two pairs of pants, a shirt, three socks, and one shoe, but on the positive, gained somebody's jacket named Joshua. I swear it looked like "Scott".

I thought about this as I labelled Maureen's clothes when she first went into memory care. Maureen had this tendency to take a jacket off and set it down. Without a name, it would go to the next person that picks it up—free clothes. They also advised me that if residents do not close their doors they might receive "shoppers". "Look! A sale in Maureen's room."

As the doting husband, I tried to mark all her clothing before we arrived, but I forgot to bring several items, which I realized only after arriving. I collected more and then realized she needed a few new items, and bought more. I then realized she had too many items and removed some. Next I realized that summer had shifted to fall and she needed warmer clothes. I was slowly creating my own rotating department store for Maureen.

Somewhere in the middle of this fun, I came to realize that using a fabric marker on her clothes and clothing tags would not always work. It did not show up on darker clothes, and writing on tags often made the name too small to read. As a man with limited domestic skills, I shopped for answers.

I remembered how my mom would iron patches on the knees of my jeans typically after I would do something that started with, "Watch this!" I discovered white iron-on patches—apparently basic knowledge for those in the garment industry. Some even come customized with names. I thought, "I will write her name on these patches and iron them into her clothing." Marking all those clothes, I wrote her name a lot. It reminded me of detention after school, writing "I will not chew gum in class" hundreds of times.

With the clothes now at the memory center, I took the material and iron to her place, figuring I would set up shop and get it all done. I timed it while they showered Maureen and the staff got her dressed so I could get it done quickly. With no space in her small room for this assembly line production, I took all her clothes into a side sitting room, plugged in the iron, and started in earnest.

Soon I had a resident lady come by and stop and watch me. I looked up and said, "Hello". She looked bewildered and said, "I've never seen that."

I asked, "What?"

"A man ironing," she said.

"Oh well, just you know…" I trailed off, hoping she would lose interest and leave. She did but came back with three more ladies—all in their eighties to nineties. I now had a small crowd amazed at the ironing man (no relation to Iron Man). They started giving me pointers. I tried hurrying so as to end the spectacle. Tags flying, some upside down, many crooked, etc.

"It's still wrinkled," one advised.

"Well, I am just doing name tags," I explained.

"Well why wouldn't you iron them too?" another asked.

I did not have a good answer, and just said, "Well, I'm in a hurry."

I might as well have said that I disliked children and puppies. I got several "Hmmfps" and they shuffled off.

I returned all the clothes to Maureen's room as the staff finished dressing her. She had missed the entire circus. However, since we walked up and down the halls several times a day, I would occasionally hear two ladies talking to each other, "He doesn't iron very well."

My wife would hear that and ask, "Who?"

"Oh, I don't know honey," I would reply.

It served as a reminder for Christmas: label any new clothes at home. It would prove easier on my reputation.

Sadly, I did not plan adequately for some things. Maureen had lost weight, so her wedding ring and another favorite would slip off easily at home. While well, she never took them off her fingers. With FTD, she sometimes took them off and set them down in places. Just before the move, I picked them up off a table and simply put them away. The gold cross necklace that she received from her father on her sixteenth birthday had never ever come off, so I thought it could stay. No. It went missing after about six weeks in the facility, in a specific three-hour window. Maureen's mother had visited in that time frame, so I never knew if she removed it for safe-keeping and simply would not tell me (I asked) or whether coincidentally it just got lost in that time. I looked everywhere. It broke my heart. I thought if I found it, I would tuck it away for the grandkids. I never did. Maureen did not seem to notice it was missing.

She never mentioned the rings either, save for once early on in the facility. While she always saw me as a safe person and someone that loved her, and would light up when I came in, she had stopped using my name many months before. She would also slip in and out of recognizing us as husband and wife. She studied my hand one time with my wedding ring.

"That?" she asked.

"My ring?" I tried to prompt.

"Yeah?" she continued.

"That's my wedding ring. We're married." I explained.

"You are?" she puzzled.

"Yes…to you." I could see the wheels turning. She looked at her hand with no ring and back at mine. I had gone too far in the explanation. She threw my hand down and got very upset but could not verbalize why. I took my ring off and stuck it in my pocket and reached for her hand.

"I have go…have to go." She stood up and started to leave. To talk her down, I redirected rather than trying to stop her.

"Would you like a snack?" I asked.

"No. She…is going."

"It's sunny outside. Would you like to walk?"

"Yes," she replied curtly.

I then guided her to the secured courtyard. I opened the door for her as I had done our whole lives together. She stepped outside. "May I walk with you?" I asked.

Just like that, her demeanor changed. She smiled and said, "Yeah" and let me take her hand. The rings never came up again.

Her knowledge of the steps required to accomplish things had almost completely deteriorated. She needed full-on assistance now. On the rare occasion, she would use the restroom herself, but I noticed one time she came out of the restroom with her hands wet. I took her back to dry them but noticed no water in the sink. She had washed them in the toilet. Steps had broken down. With nothing more than, "Honey. Let's wash our hands here in the sink together," she did so willingly. Lecturing, scolding, or correcting would have caused her to spiral and would have accomplished nothing.

She also still paced and burned so much weight, although she seemed to have light meals regularly.

In the mornings, I would bring her Starbucks to have with her breakfast. Her go-to had evolved over the years to a grande, soy, 185 degree, no foam, no water, one pump vanilla chai tea latte. As her FTD progressed, the extra hot dropped off. While she could not ask for them by name or remember their ingredients, she would smile at the cup and say, "Ooooh, I just love these... "

In the evenings, I always asked staff how she had eaten. She usually ate some of her dinner with help, but occasionally not at all. When the staff failed to get her to eat, they would wrap it and stick it in their fridge. I would have them reheat it. I sat with her a bit and got her excited about eating, and then they brought it back out, and she ate it all. This typically happened twice a week.

Back at the garage and behind the scenes, I wrote out a quick informal will for myself, but I needed to do a real one when funds allowed. I left it in an obvious spot on my desk in the garage with a copy to my sister. If I suddenly passed in the middle of the night and someone found me later, they would see this paper signed by me and know what to do, who to call, and our last wishes. Most importantly, where to find funds to take care of Maureen—what I called project manager preparations, or just the actions of a smitten husband.

I took her out of the facility any time she felt up to it. The outings did get harder. Restaurants became a no-go. She would get too agitated by the time the meal arrived, so I had them immediately box it. I took to bringing her some barbeque pulled pork from her favorite place. We would sit in one of the side dining rooms and ate together in general quiet. Noise and unfamiliar settings could really set her off. At those times, she acted trapped, like she needed to escape.

While we did have troubles, that facility had mostly great people. They put on a carnival and seasonal parties with pleasant, light activities and fun food. Maureen kind of went in and out of them. She would do a few minutes, but then wanted to walk around away from it, and then would come back. Combatting the stimuli everywhere, I kept her pretty even-tempered by moving her in and out of it—we danced. I would lead her and move her to the rhythm of her mood. Sometimes I guessed wrong. Sometimes I had her lead and watched for her cues and then followed. In that way, we danced daily.

At the carnival, she lobbed some bean bags, tossed a ping pong ball, and we got our photo taken with red noses on. I spread out each of these activities. She tried some popcorn, licorice, animal crackers, and punch. She liked the animal crackers a lot. She got tired a couple hours in.

No sooner did I pull her to a quiet place to begin the calming than her son came for a surprise visit with the granddaughters. While Maureen normally loved their visits, the carnival already had her highly stimulated. Sadly, the visit only lasted about twenty minutes before she started getting really agitated. She started using the word "crap" and I knew more colorful words would start coming quickly as she escalated. FTD steals someone's filter. We scooted the girls out so they did not have to witness any sort of meltdown of their grandma at the ages of eleven and nine.

I figured they could handle it, but I wanted them to have happy memories of their Grandma Maureen. Outside, I explained to the girls that Grandma had a permanent sickness and had a hard time figuring out how to do things. She got confused and frustrated a lot, and the people here took good care of her. What else could I say? I left their father to fill in what he thought appropriate and asked him to let me know ahead of visits so I could try and get her in a good mood first.

The next weekend, I thought I would try taking Maureen to Multnomah Falls, as the memory facility had waterfall murals in the halls we walked together. She said she would like to go. Unfortunately, I did not realize they now had a shuttle service, so you cannot park right there in the lot unless you get there really early. She did not do well waiting in the lot for the bus, getting on the bus, or sitting on the bus. She wanted to leave. She looked at the falls only briefly. Other than a brief smile, she could not enjoy herself. She kept looking for a way to escape—not really running off, just eyes searching and worried. I came to realize that perhaps I had imposed her old self onto her new self. I could not keep chasing our old lifestyle. She needed it all lowkey. I failed at reading her that day.

I brought her back and kissed and hugged her goodbye, but she pushed me away. Understandably, the outing had made her angry and confused.

I went back to the garage of our old home and had a good cry. I loved her so much but struggled to figure out how to keep us dancing. She got angry more often now. I was running low on energy and options but rallied again. I thought, "I'll keep trying. She is so worth it. I love you baby."

The days and weeks blurred into each other.

Three months had gone by and there were still no bites on the house.

I kept working full-time but flex time, so I still saw Maureen every day, two to three times per day.

I still lived in the garage on the couch, but that was taking its toll on my sleep. Winter would come, and I would need to find another solution to the cold garage.

I received some support in a network that I stumbled across, the Association for Frontotemporal Degeneration. I applied to their closed group and got accepted. They had a strong collection of FTD sufferers and caregivers. The administrator kept things non-judgmental, supportive, and interactive. I found myself reading their content a lot and eventually writing a lot too. It helped in my down times.

Near the end of October, I took one night over to Cannon Beach alone—our beach: the first time I had slept in a bed in nearly three months. I just needed twenty-four hours to recharge. I wandered up and down the streets and sat quietly on the beach reading Hemingway's *The Old Man and the Sea*. Other than ordering food and checking in and out, I said nothing to anyone. While the bed felt nice and afforded me that good night's sleep, I remained too anxious and headed back mid-morning to check on Maureen. I missed her.

Each week, I shopped for her and kept her well supplied in absorbent underwear, wipes, Ensure, and snacks. I would bring her chai teas three to four times per week.

I changed out the decorations in her room and on her door once a month for the holidays or seasons. I used a Hawaiian theme for August, then moved to a pleasant fall, then to Halloween (playful, not scary), and then November into Thanksgiving. I wanted her to feel like she had a context, a frame of reference in the world. I never knew whether it mattered or not, but I would point out familiar decorations from our home, and she would smile. Her name and her photos in the curio box on the wall outside her room always stayed the same so she could find her way. However, she rarely did that unassisted.

We had pleasant weather that fall. As such, I tried taking her on another drive to the Oregon beach. I knew it had always been a favorite of hers in the past. She loved the beach. We discussed it, and she genuinely seemed interested. I thought she wanted to get out. Sadly, it proved a disaster. I packed her up, and we got some breakfast and her soy chai. We started down the road, and things seemed ok for a while, but halfway there, they went downhill. The negativity and nastiness kicked in. I contemplated turning the car around but thought maybe it would pass. It did not. I think we spent ninety minutes at Cannon Beach. Despite my best efforts at redirecting, it seemed obvious FTD's grip simply would not let her come out of that negative spiral. We started the long drive back.

As much as it pained me, I realized that at least at this point in the disease, she could no longer do outings that lasted over an hour. FTD had left her with a limited capacity for travel and waiting. Perhaps, I thought, when she fell deeper into the dementia (I did not wish that, but just knew it would happen), she might not struggle and get frustrated as much. She might become less torn between what she knows and can comprehend.

On the drive there, I tried to use soothing talk with her, yet she fired off things like "I'm gonna kill you," and "I hate you." She told me five minutes earlier that she loved me. I treated these barbs like mere soft needles—no real damage was done. Dementia can cause a person to spiral like that but can also loosen its grip for just a random moment. She would have a few moments here and there where she seemed lucid—fleeting but definitely there.

That fall, she would say as we sat together, "I am scared. I am just terrified." However, I could not get much more out of her. I did not think anything at the facility scared her (i.e. a caregiver or other resident). I think she genuinely understood in those moments that she kept losing her mental grip. She would say, "This is all wrong. I don't understand. It scares me." She would then come out of it again. This happened maybe once or twice a week. I shared these types of things with the head nurse and director, so they too could monitor her.

She would mention death periodically. "This is just death. I'm gonna just die." She typically said this during her rage spells, so I never knew for sure how deeply she meant it. However, one very poignant morning, she said very sorrowfully for the first time, "I don't want to die. I don't want to die." I held back tears and told her I did not want her to die either, and I asked her why she thought that. She could only say "It's too much." She then went back into the dementia again.

Occasionally in the early evening, while she seemed genuinely happy to see me, she would interestingly make the comment that she sometimes got upset and did not know why. That sounded telling and powerful to know that she could look back and reflect on that.

I told her not to worry of course, and that I knew she loved me. She sometimes professed that she did.

These kinds of things obviously saddened me tremendously and made my heart hurt for my wife Maureen. She must have frequently wrestled in her mind with the dementia and those moments of realization. However, quite literally 99% of the time, I heard none of this—just random words and pacing.

She remained loving with good moments too. Sometimes we just sat on this brown couch sort of on the edge of the activity but not in the middle of it. She liked to just sit there on the edge and people watch, drinking her drink and holding my hand on the couch. I loved those moments too. On occasion, she would tell me that she loved me unprompted. That made me feel pretty wonderful.

Often, she let me lie next to her and listen to music. However, figuring out steps continued to challenge her. At night when I came in and they had already laid her down, she would start drifting off. I saw her slippers under her head like a pillow sometimes—an uncomfortable pillow for certain. I would swap them with her actual pillow, and she would wake up. I would kiss her gently and tell her that I just moved her pillow to make her more comfortable. I had no reason to point out the errors. FTD kept her from self-correcting and learning anyway. It made her unlearn. I just kept things positive.

"Thank you," she would say. "I I don't...I...why I'm upset...I..."

"No worries. I love you and always will."

"Love love love too," she would push out best she could. She would then go on with a collection of words that made no sense and start to drift off again.

With her eyes closed, I would kiss her and tell her I would bring her a chai in the morning, and she would whisper ok. Then I would leave.

I still took her on outings when the weather cooperated but kept them simple: for example, to the park with a milkshake and her playlist. I had shifted and tried to keep things all lowkey, but it still tore at me. I asked myself often if I did enough for her. I did not want her to feel ignored or sad. I did not want her to die and not have felt loved 'till the very end. Not every resident there had visitors.

Two people in her facility died in that first few months. They kept it really quiet so residents would not dwell on it. I thought that they must have understood that a person had died—wouldn't they? Maureen never mentioned it. A frail woman of similar build as Maureen, but about twenty years her senior, had died first. I had seen her a couple of times but did not know much about her and never saw her with any visitors. They typically wheeled her in and out on a reclining chair they called a Geri-Chair. The other gentleman that died had spent most of his career as a Seaman. He had a lot of character—a bit of a troublemaker in one of those good ways that made you laugh. Both deaths occurred suddenly. They remained ever-present in my mind—the fleeting nature of life.

Generally, Maureen had little pain. Sadly though, when she had a pain, she could not point to it or verbalize where. Her stomach seemed fine. Her leg swelling had left. However, random pains still emerged occasionally.

She still got thin as hell. I think in November she dropped to one hundred pounds even. She paced constantly, so any calories she took in, she burned. She kept drinking the Ensure, but her eating remained sporadic. My frustration with the facility, even after multiple discussions, centered on the fact that they simply put the meals in front of her. She would get up and walk away due to her anxiety, and they would just let her.

She would sit for a couple of bites and then get up again. I would try different ways and places to get her to sit down. I would try taking a break and coming back to it. I tried eating with her—me taking extra small bites. I tried bringing her other food—the things she liked. We had mixed results, so I kept trying. One night, they served a good fattening dinner (presumably as a precursor to Thanksgiving later that month) of meatloaf with gravy and some sort of cheesy potato dish. I had to work really hard to get her to eat about half before she simply got done.

She became irritable most days, though she always greeted me sweetly. It could turn fast though! She still asked if I came to take her home. She still asked if I would sleep there. I continued to struggle internally with both. I kept saying, "This is our home. I just sleep in a different bed at night." She eventually became more accepting of these ideas.

We still had some tremendously tender moments. She did love to see me come in. She did like to hold my hand and give me hugs and kisses. She smiled at me a lot. She would say "come with me" and grab my hand. I would stand up and then…she would not walk. She did not know where to go. I suggested down the hall or her room or outside if the weather looked nice, and she would say, "Ok" and lead the way.

As I held her hand while we walked, I would tell her, "I will always love you."

In one of her more thoughtful moments, she replied, "I hope so, or I'll be gone." She said it in a looking-off manner as if to imply that my love existed as the only thing, the last thing, that still gave her some meaning. I worried that she feared that she would simply disappear for everyone and not matter anymore. But maybe she did not think on such things…maybe.

I tried changing things up to keep her engaged. I looked at love poems and saw an Elizabeth Barrett Browning one that I had read to her many times when we were dating. She liked it. "How do I love thee? Let me count the ways…" Sadly, her attention span had all but vanished. I could no longer read to her without her getting up and walking away.

FTD keeps attention diverted in multiple directions. Their mind simply races and does not know how to put the brakes on anymore. She just needed some calm to quiet the pacing. We used music to help with that. Like everything, it worked until it did not.

People think those with dementia have their minds just stop working. No. Their minds work constantly, so much that they have too much noise in their head. They lose the ability to gauge, to filter, to prioritize. It churns more than it ever has perhaps—it's very overwhelming. That, perhaps, better captures her dementia.I simply loved Maureen and did not want her hurting or confused anymore. But my wants felt unanswered. I just prayed she knew I would love her 'till the very end and never felt alone. However, sadly, I had a certification trip for work, which would take me out of town for three days—the first and only days I would not spend with her in the care facility. I had to prepare.

I did not want her to feel abandoned, as she had needed many reassurances since her move. She actually needed them most of the years that I knew her, but recently more so. We walked and talked quite a bit. She worried periodically, even with the FTD, like she had done something wrong or that she got "broken" as she said. I reminded her often, "You are good. You are smart. You are special." She seemed calmed by that. I had to reinforce her worth, as she did not get much of that in her early and mid-life years.

I did not want these efforts to go backwards in the three days of this required trip.

I downloaded ten photos of me to a digital picture frame set as a slide show and placed it on her nightstand to loop continuously for the three days. I held signs in the photos that included phrases like "You are smart", "You are good and kind", "You are loved", and so forth.

I also pre-wrote three love letters, placed them in envelopes, and asked a caregiver to read one a day to her—short letters with a picture of us together and simple messages: I miss you, the words of reassurance, and I will come home soon.

Lastly, I called her each evening. Though her focus made those calls last less than a minute, she heard my voice and seemed to recognize it somehow.

When I returned home, I went to her (with a chai tea latte of course), and she smiled, happy to see me. She did not behave like, "Where have you been?" The passage of time had become hard for her to grasp—the joy of this story. My worries proved unnecessary, but the preparation kept us close. We walked and talked, and she stayed in good spirits as though I had never left. That relieved me so much, but I also never let another day go by again where I did not see her. I placed that expectation on myself, whether right or wrong.

The staff started doing a better job in the evenings and over-all. Maureen's emotional crashes became much less frequent in November and throughout the next year, reverting primarily to just the communication and eating struggles.

However, I did get surprised after an informal conversation about potentially trying a mood stabilizing drug. They had started her on it three days before I found out. Their policy of notifying me ahead of time failed. They had put her on Mirtazapine. Again, I knew we had decided to try something, and had discussed Mirtazapine. However, we had not yet settled on anything. We had planned to have a conference call in a couple of days between Parkview, me, and her primary care physician to discuss it. This did not happen. I wrote to Parkview and expressed my concern, but I also forgave them, as communication had proven a constant battle. I also knew Mirtazapine had risen to the top as the tamest drug to try anyway.

They spoke of an additional emergency mood drug if Maureen got really out of sorts, and I emphatically said no. I did not want Plan B to become Plan A—as that would be easiest for staff. Besides, I had seen an improvement in her mood, as had the day-to-day caregivers. She resisted less. Things started levelling out a bit. I watched closely for side effects and requested that Parkview do the same.

Maureen seldom had outbursts anymore. When she did, they seemed more out of her confusion about steps. I still chose to put her pajamas on some nights myself. Some nights she still resisted a lot, but eventually we got them on. If she already had clean and dry underwear, that helped—it meant less "messing" with her. I could now often tell when she wanted to sit on the bed for a while and not lie down. Eventually, she would mellow, and I would ask again for her to lie down with me. I would play a couple of songs, and we would just lie there together on her tiny twin bed until she fell asleep. I enjoyed those times. She would hold my hand, and she seemed to have such peace.

They say caregivers need to take care of themselves too. As I mentioned before, while caregivers typically agree with that statement, they also typically ask, "When exactly do I do that?" I tried.

In the previous two and a half years of caring for her, I stress-ate and gained forty pounds. Trying to keep the house spotless for a sale, I ate a lot of takeout. I signed up for a cheap gym membership that came with a trainer to guide my workouts and nutrition. Open twenty-four hours, I had no excuses. With the special, it wasn't a huge hit on my already struggling financial situation. Me getting sick, or worse, would not help Maureen at all.

I started to gradually change what I ate and got smart about finding the right foods and easy ways to prepare it, and I would take it to work with me. My promise to Maureen years ago to live two weeks longer than her so as to take care of her through the end would not come to fruition unless I started taking better care of myself.

I helped Maureen navigate her environment best I could, but her inability to convey a narrative or explain herself challenged the caregivers. Once, a caregiver came up to her while she was pacing mid-day because she looked a little more worried than usual.

Very kindly she asked, "Maureen, honey, do you need something?"

Maureen looked at her and asked, "Where's my baby?"

Alzheimer's patients will often cling to a period in their life, perhaps decades earlier, but will remember it in vivid detail. For women, that might often focus on their time as young mothers caring for infants. Most care facilities have a few dolls on hand that they can provide to these patients to help calm them.

The caregiver, trained in Alzheimer's but not in FTD, took Maureen to a side room and said, "We have babies in here."

She handed Maureen one of the dolls that had quite messy hair. Maureen looked at the doll and laughably said, "She's ugly," and tossed her down.

The caregiver asked, "You don't like her?"

After a long pause, Maureen replied, "Where's my baby?" and walked out of the room. She walked toward one of the med-aids familiar to her. "I, I, I...want my baby."

The med-aid looked at the caregiver, and the caregiver replied, "I tried to give her one of the babies, but she didn't want it."

Around that time, I came into the grand room and called Maureen's name.

She turned toward me with her arms raised for a hug and said, "Yeah. My, my, my baby." The staff started to laugh, and I had no idea why 'till they recounted the story later.

As noted, her kids would come up when other events brought them to town. I made myself scarce so they could have some one-on-one time. It sounded like it went fine usually, but they often said they found it difficult to understand what Maureen talked about. I frequently told them about Maureen's condition and her word salad. Whenever they told me they planned on coming up, I would try to coach them ahead of the visits. But it seemed they approached the visits like they knew their mom and did not need the coaching, so I backed off.

I do not think they really knew their current mother—even before the FTD. They remembered the mom of their youth. They would come up to town when they had something else going on and needed a place to crash—rarely just to visit. I remembered numerous times that we came down for all sorts of kid things and holidays. We would try to sit each of the kids and grandkids down to hear everything going on in their lives. We craved those few minutes of one-on-one with them. You really get to know someone when you actually take the time to listen to them. Years earlier, Maureen had made the comment that she thought she would perpetually be their "mom" to them and not a person—likely a relationship issue for many families.

I still regularly took her to her mother's apartment for coffee most Thursdays. Maureen never said much and would go completely quiet after little less than an hour. Maureen would just get "done". She never talked about these visits. She responded with, "Yeah, Mom wants that." Apathy often comes with FTD.

Her mother still did not understand how to engage Maureen, but at almost ninety, she never would—which was not her fault. She loved Maureen deeply no doubt, but her habit of talking "a mile a minute" about her own life and/or probing for something she thought she should know about yours, proved disengaging for Maureen. The moment you tried to answer, her mother would start up again. You could not finish a thought before her mother leapt in on what she herself had done better or longer or harder or...It proved a challenge for me to keep up with the conversation as a healthy person. With the communication challenges of FTD, Maureen found it impossible. These coffees became increasingly difficult to keep going or to justify. Perhaps I had just stretched myself too thin. Maureen usually got nothing out of the coffees. I did them for her mother, and it took her mom 'till near the end of Maureen's illness to understand that.

Her friends seldom came to visit. They all had their own lives, but I also saw two other issues influencing that (common for many friends and families the world over). First, they did not know what to do or how to act. It startled them to see their dear friend confused or lashing out—completely not herself. When Maureen remained calm and wanted to walk with her friends, they had to help her along as they might an elderly parent, but as their friend of the same age. Her loving and caring friends just found themselves in uncertain waters. I saw it written across many of their faces: "How do we relate? What do we say?" I would explain as I did with her family, "Just spend time with her. Just let her know she is loved.

Just be reaffirming." Second, I think they just wanted to remember Maureen the way she had lived before all this.

People with dementia have not stopped living. They deserve the same loving attention and support that we all do. They still have a life of joy and sadness. Do not forget them before their time.

Separately, Maureen still occasionally said she wanted me to take her home. She had this sense of "where do you go?" when I left her each day. On an outing, I took her to the old house where I still lived in the garage. I had moved a mattress up to a room as the winter cold set in. The house had still not sold, so I hoped for a spring blitz. I showed Maureen the couch that I had slept on in the garage. I showed her all the items, still packed. I showed her the emptiness of the rest of the house. She took it in. She did not act startled or sad. Things felt familiar. I explained again that we needed to sell the house for money so we could continue to support things like her medical care—not in a blaming way, just helping her to understand. She had a moment of clarity and hugged me and said, "Thank you". She seemed ok when we left, and while she asked about home a couple of times after, that too subsided.

Sometimes Maureen seemed downright depressed. We would sit in one of the side activity rooms on the couch. She would get a little agitated and sad.

Once, after a lot of ambiguous statements like trying to explain something, she said, "I just want to be me." So powerful. All single syllable words. No words over four letters. All words she could still regularly use. She found a way to string them together to tell me she knew that she couldn't feel, act, or do things the way that she used to. I said, "I know baby. I know." I held her tight.

I bought a fridge for her room. It had a window so she could see into it for the rare times that she initiated action. It was really small but large enough to hold a few of her Fantas. I knew clutter was an issue for her mind.

She had developed more of a sweet tooth over the last few months. She happened upon orange Fanta and really took to it, to the point of looking for it. Several months prior, we had started with cans, but the mechanics became too complicated. I would find cans with no tabs on top, as she had ripped them off trying to open them. We went to plastic screw-top bottles that worked well but proved too big, and she spilled a lot. This upset her. After placing her in the care facility, I found one store that carried the tiny twelve-ounce plastic bottles. She liked to screw the cap on and unscrew it again. Those worked well. I kept her stocked with Fantas, along with yogurts and fruit. I kept other snacks in a wicker basket on her nightstand. She liked small cookies like Milanos or chocolate chip. In her early days at the care facility, when she could still initiate those activities, I would find cookies in her room, opened and partially eaten. I would also include a little gum. Oh, how she loved to chew gum. I of course monitored this closely, as swallowing problems can occur later in the progression of FTD. When swallowing looked at all labored, the gum would stop. Truly, all unsupervised snacking would have to stop. Oddly, Maureen lost her ability to initiate opening a snack before any swallowing issues, so it never caused concern.

She had also developed a passion for Altoids—perhaps due to the intense flavor. The peppermint ones came in a red box, and I would keep one in the console of the car. When I took her on outings, I would help her into the car and buckle her seatbelt. She would eye the Altoids and make for them even before I could get around to the driver side. It always made me laugh.

They come in a hinged box, and I would watch as she struggled to open it. She did not understand which way to hold the box. I tried not to step in until some time had passed, but would then offer to help. She would say no and keep struggling, but would eventually get it open and become frustrated at herself if she spilled them. I found the tin did not have a traditional hinge, rather just cut tabs. When alone, I lifted the lid and gave a tug. The lid came off, and I bent back in the tabs and returned the lid. Now the lid was removable, not hinged. On the next trip, she saw the Altoids and went for them again. She opened the box easily because it no longer mattered from which direction she pulled. You could see the grin as she had figured it out. From that day on, I modified all tins before she saw them. To this day, I still do that as a remembrance.

As an FTD caregiver, search for those little things that make your loved one's life easier. It requires you to become an observer of human nature. I suggest these tips:

1. Watch closely what they struggle with and challenge yourself to take away the struggle for next time—but not in that moment. They will figure it out the next time and be thrilled with themselves rather than feel like you "took it from them."

2. Discover how they drink and remove the obstacles. If they like to pull lids off, give them a juice box with the straw already in it when they see it. If they throw things, get children's sippy cups in simple colors and not characters (leave them their dignity). Transfer drinks to easy-to-use containers.

3. Do not just rely on what they tell you verbally but watch for visual cues. I looked for flush cheeks, not waiting for her to tell me she was hot.

4. Watch for obsessive compulsive behavior—often a sign there is a crash coming or even in progress.

5. Follow their eyes. They will point to what they want more times than not. They serve as good prompts for you to try things.

6. Most importantly, talk to them, not about them. This will keep them engaged even when you think they are not. Do not abandon conversation, just arm yourself with more tools.

You have to notice the nuances. You make the adjustments. However, you must remain vigilant. Those adjustments will not work the next week or the next day, and you will need to adjust again, even further. That describes the commitment of a caregiver. You are in it for the long-term. It can make you weary, but it is a privilege to be the one they trust most.

Maureen liked short outings for a soy chai and croissant. We would go to the drive-up and stay in the car—that seemed easiest. We would sit there and talk a little, listening to the radio and just enjoying a simple time. I would take her back and we would walk in the facility for a while and sit and talk some more. I would play music from her playlist, and we would sway-dance, and, if it seemed alright, I would give her a little spin. I would bring fresh flowers every week. We had our routine. Struggles still remained, but I took from it only what I chose to.

Mid-November on a Friday night, when helping to change her, I noticed a hard spot to the right of her abdomen and below the waistline. I showed Mary, the site RN, and she decided to get Maureen back on a stool softener to make sure she did not have a blockage. I wrote Dr. Da Graca to get an opinion as well. He said not to worry but also suggested a visual check-up. The tumor might have just gotten denser and would do nothing more—it was hard to say. It bothered her from time to time but not constantly. I noticed when she rubbed it, and we monitored it 'till the appointment.

I finished changing her, put on some music, and stood there holding her as I often did. She enjoyed "Calling on Angels" by Michael Allen Harrison and Haley Johnsen. She would say, "Oooh...one one... my favorites." A little bit into the music, she once said, "You should be with me all the time." I loved those moments. If we could have afforded for me to retire, I WOULD have been "with her all the time."

With her condition stable and just before Thanksgiving, I decided to try an overnight at the old house. Since I still lived in the garage, I brought a small table and two chairs for upstairs and pre-bought her favorite barbeque and ice cream. I made the mattress up with the wet-proof cover and a full sheet set as opposed to just my standard comforter thrown on top. I put a few of her Fantas in the fridge.

I picked her up around 3:30 p.m. and took two changes of everything plus wipes, depends, toothbrush, and the Mirtazapine (mood) and Melatonin (sleep), and a couple of Ensures. I hoped I had us covered. We then went to the old house. It went pretty well. She wandered a bit, perhaps just to check things out. We worked our way through dinner with a few "up and wanders". She liked the ice cream. She got tired early, so I gave her the Mirtazapine and Melatonin, and we listened to a couple of songs and held each other. I helped her on with her pajamas with only a little resistance and then settled into bed early. She slept a little restlessly, but we made it through the night. I watched her sleep. It felt so good to sleep next to my wife again.

The next morning, we got up early and got her dressed. The hard spot on her stomach had turned red and it worried me. I got her to brush her teeth and her hair by herself by placing the tooth- and hairbrush in her hand and coaching her. I decided to push my luck and take her to a new breakfast place I found—something small, quiet, and basic. I thought that would go over well. It did, sort of. She never felt totally comfortable and only picked at her breakfast.

I called that overnighter a success, and it encouraged me to try more in the future. However, the next day we had our appointment with Dr. Da Graca regarding the hardening in her right abdomen. The prognosis made me feel helpless. He could not provide any recommendations given her condition and dementia. He had no confidence that she would survive ANY surgery. If she did, the anesthesia would make her permanently non-responsive afterwards. He knew the hardening came from the tumors. He referred us to a scan from June, but he did not see a need yet for a new one. He said the tumors sat in the safest spot, but I knew we could not call anywhere truly safe.

He liked seeing her pace in the exam room. He liked that she still moved a lot. I explained that she rarely experienced pain. While pleased with that, the doctor prepared me that the tumors could eventually press on her stomach and intestines. This would create a blockage and potentially lacerate them. When that happened, she would quickly come to "her end", as he put it. Normally he could explore options or reroutes and add an ostomy bag requiring daily cleaning, but, again, she could not have surgery. Her condition would also make a bag completely impractical anyway—she would never understand or learn not to tug on it.

I said she had fairly regular bowel movements, which made him happy. He expressed the importance of keeping that moving and clear. He recommended reaching out to the palliative care team regarding pain management if that developed later.

With a lump in my throat, I asked about her time. He said he had no idea. She could have months before something critical happened. I asked about years. He said he could not say that and did not want to raise my expectations.

This crushed me as I stared at my beautiful wife pacing and holding my hand.

He said, "When it happens, it will happen fast."

We had no options. He said they did not even use chemo for this type of cancer as it proved ineffective and would make her really sick. She could not afford to get sick and lose even more weight.

While Maureen's dementia safeguarded her from dwelling on these issues, I simply felt lost. Would the FTD take her first, or the cancer? The FTD had progressed at a much more rapid pace than anything I had read in articles or papers or in the AFTD support group. Would the two issues continue to work against each other? Every day added more questions than answers.

I wrote and told her kids and mother that weekend to let them know. I had this dread that the end would come soon.

I decided to treat the upcoming Christmas season like her last. I wanted to make sure she had joy in her favorite time of year. I loved my baby so much. Thank God the FTD seemed to mask any worry on her part. Maureen's occasional lucid moments seemed far fewer now. I could shoulder that worry alone.

I started playing her favorite Christmas songs on my phone as we walked—integrating them into her playlist. She hummed and lightly sang along. I played the Trans-Siberian Orchestra's Christmas Canon and Faith Hill's "Where are you Christmas?" for her. She had always called this canon one of her favorite piano pieces and loved the combination with the children's voices. She found that sound utterly pleasant. Faith Hill's song from the live-action Grinch movie brought back memories from seeing it on our honeymoon. We watched it every anniversary, so the song had stayed with her. Also a big Elvis Presley fan, she always grinned at his rendition of Winter Wonderland.

We would sit together, and then she would stand up abruptly, as she often got restless. Sometimes I would give her a light hug around her waist while I was still sitting. She would lean down and kiss the top of my head—great moments. Sometimes she would lightly rub my upper back. She understood our bond.

Sometimes the exchanges would make me laugh. I would say, "I love you." She would reply, "That's true." I would profess, "I will always love you." Matter-of-factly, she answered, "Yes you will."

I would rub and scratch her back a lot, as her skin got very dry. I tried to get her to drink water whenever possible to get her and her skin more hydrated. I also rubbed lotion on her back. She reacted well as long as I prepared her for that initial shock of a little cold. I got better as time went on by holding the lotion in my closed hand a bit first to warm it up.

When you see your time together fading, you cannot help but think back to your first times together. I thought of our first date movie, *Jerry Maguire*, and downloaded Springsteen's "Secret Garden". I played it while we were sitting on the couch in the Tulip Hall (she resided in the neighboring Daffodil Hall). I asked her if she remembered the song.

"Yes," she smiled. "I love, just love...I've not...this long time."

I stood her up and we slow danced, or just kind of swayed back and forth to the song. I lifted her hand and lightly twirled her once around and then came back together. She beamed. A staff member came by for something. I saw her through the reflection in the window. She smiled and turned around and left us to dance alone.

I had made music the constant for my wife. Her mood, verbalization, and physicality shifted frequently, but when I put on a song she knew, a calm came over her, often accompanied by her humming. When she allowed me, we stood and danced or just swayed. Her demeanor would soften, and she would rest her hands and head on me as if to say, "This is good. This is right. This is my joy."

When I was alone, I cried a lot those days—still do. I started missing her already, which I knew I needed to try and stop doing. They call it ambiguous grief. I found my eyes watering as we sat together listening to music, talking or even holding hands. I found it harder and harder to push that down and focus on joyful experiences with her.

Nobody had ever loved me so much as she did. Maureen gave me the gift of a bottomless heart. That season when I asked, "Do you want to see the decorations at the mall?" She replied, "...be with you." She had told me that many times in our life together. It never failed to touch my soul. It touched me the deepest of anything.

I found myself coming by early in the morning to watch her sleep—to see her awaken and still lying in bed. I would give her a smile, a kiss, a hug, and brush the hair from her face. She smiled so wide in the morning, delighted to see me. Caregiving staff commented too that she typically woke in the morning so happy and content. I hated to go to work.

I tried the care facility's in-person monthly support group a couple times. While worth the effort, I left disappointed. The lady presented some bits from Teepa Snow, an authority on dementia, that I always find entertaining and insightful. However, the presenter talked to us like professional caregivers in a training seminar, not as the family of our loved ones. She explained signs to tell if your loved one had dementia, but everyone there knew their loved one had dementia—hence the group. We all had experienced it for a while and had developed workarounds with our loved ones. I had hoped they would provide this as more of a Q&A or sharing session. I stopped going.

Her son and his new wife came for Thanksgiving, as their exes had the kids that year. I made a formal dinner reservation for one of the rooms—removed from the busyness. I knew Maureen would like that better.

I decorated her unit for Christmas a day earlier than planned so her son could see it and Maureen got to experience it longer. I did not know how long I had left with her. She loved Christmas so much.

I found a thin but tall flocked artificial tree perfect for Maureen's small room, however, they had sold out. I forced them to sell me the floor model. Since they had it assembled already and it threatened to rain, I brought it over, put it up, and plugged it in her room that same night, just so she could see it. She beamed with delight.

Thanksgiving morning, I got there early before she woke up and changed her decorations outside her room. After she awoke, I decorated the inside of her room, and she helped me hang ornaments on the tree. It looked really cute. We placed many of her snow people and snow globes around the room. She smiled and studied them. She gently touched each one ever so cautiously, like treasures. I watched carefully to make sure she did not get overwhelmed. I could put some back in the boxes, but she seemed to delight in it all.

Thanksgiving dinner itself did not really go well. Her son and his wife arrived, and we did get a quieter side room. However, the noise from all the other residents' families really agitated Maureen. She would not eat more than a few bites. While happy to see her son, it did not end up as successful as we had hoped. That happens, and you have to stay nimble.

Her mild abdominal discomfort turned into periodic pain, so I spoke to the palliative care team and got some pain meds for her that next morning: Hydrocodone. Over the next several days, there did not appear to be any significant side effects. They referred to it as one of the milder medications and had prescribed the smallest dosage. It helped.

The Christmas season (with some of my prodding) seemed to bring out more visitors to see Maureen. Her best friend and Matron of Honor at our wedding, Candy, came that weekend after Thanksgiving. Maureen immediately recognized her and cried, "Candace!"— beautiful to see. Another good friend, Jeanne and her sister visited a few days later, and she also seemed to recognize them. Lastly, her friend Esther and husband Steve visited. She showed less recognition but enough familiarity, even grabbing Esther's hand and walking down the halls with her. Each of these ladies had known Maureen most of their lives, since they were little girls. It made me so happy to see. Maureen, if she had any self-consciousness about her condition, never showed it. She took her friends and walked with them and talked. While mostly word salad, they could see how utterly happy they made her.

December 2nd came around—our eighteenth wedding anniversary. I prepared and set my expectations low. I brought her back to the old house to spend the night with me. Things went pretty well. She did not want to eat much, but did like her ice cream. I tried playing Grinch for her as we had done each year. However, she could no longer hold that kind of attention. I bought her new pajamas and a new watch. I had bought an inexpensive, slip-on watch like a bracelet (no clasp) with a large, visible analog face. She had always worn watches. I thought she would like the renewed familiarity, although she would not use it to tell the time. She did like the watch and studied it. She loved the ultra-soft pajamas. She slept well after going to bed early listening to a couple of her favorite songs.

In the morning we got up early, had breakfast, and went on our deferred shopping mall trip. We got there early enough in the morning so that she only had to contend with a small handful of mall walkers. With the shops still closed, we had gotten there ahead of the crowds. We had no plans to shop. I took her there to see the decorations. With her soy chai and a cranberry bliss bar, she looked content. She studied the tree, the wreaths, the lights, and all the decorations. After an hour, she got agitated, and I returned her to her facility before it became a crash. I had pushed as much as I dared.

The rest of the Christmas season, I looked for these simple joys.

AFTD Social Media Post – 12/8/18

A Gift

As the holiday season is upon us all, I know this can be a difficult time. I know it is for me. So many of our holiday traditions with our loved ones struggling with FTD have to be cancelled or compromised. It makes it hard to live the life with the rest of our family and the life with our loved one and striking that balance for them and ourselves.

Tears flow at the strangest times, and often it is because we are fatigued. I know the quality caregivers of this group are always trying to find ways of including our struggling loved ones into the holiday season when so much seems beyond their physical and mental capabilities anymore. Yes, and those goalposts keep moving, don't they?

My wife cannot do crowds anymore—I mean like a real fast crash whether in the store, restaurant, show, or anywhere. With the bustle of the season, that makes it hard to find the right venue. We keep looking though, don't we?

I lucked out here in Portland, Oregon as my wife and I love to go to the Pittock Mansion and view their antique Christmas decorations and displays. It is a 104-year-old building salvaged now as a museum tribute to that family. This has always been a highlight for my wife at this time of year. However, thousands of people go through there for the same reason.

I reached out to the facility and explained the situation, and they were very accommodating and had someone meet us there an hour before it opened to the public for a private viewing. Yes, we had a Christmas-decorated mansion for just the two of us. She enjoyed it immensely— she had few words and needed lots of help, but her smile spoke volumes.

Keep persevering caregivers, through the pain and tears to make the happy moments that you will remember and treasure long after the trials of creating those moments have faded from memory. You can do it!

We mined the season for the joys that we could.

When I had changed her into her pajamas in the evenings, I really took in how frail she had become. Down to ninety-something pounds, she sat there, a physical shadow of herself. I worried for how little time it seemed she had. We had no idea when, or if, the tumors would shift against her intestines and stomach, which would bring the end. Perhaps, instead, with the FTD, she would suddenly aspirate. I feared both possibilities as well as the others I could not yet conceive of.

That season, everyone she would have wanted to see had visited her except for maybe her dear cousin in Idaho. While her children came to see her, most of the five grandchildren did not. However, I think on it now and reckon that perhaps her kids just wanted their children to remember Maureen full of life and not frail and confused. I wanted her to see them but had to respect their wishes.

Indeed, Maureen had become frail, thin, and weak. When I changed her, I felt hard veins in parts of her legs. I suspected this related to the weight loss. She still walked, but now with a slight shake. This shake appeared sometimes when she held an object too. I had not seen this before. I would describe it less like a tremor than simply just frailty.

She still walked, ate, spoke, smiled, heard, and saw, so I remained thankful. That month, she had life and felt loved and knew me when I entered the room. I could cherish those moments as we lay together listening to music, me saying I loved her and her sometimes saying she loved me back. I called her, "My baby", and she called me her baby back, as we had done for years. I had to take that and hold it and not dwell on the future. Though the future came pretty suddenly.

Chapter 10

Our Moments

Scott's Journal – 12/20/18

My heart is very heavy, as my baby only has days or weeks to live.

I have cried so much in just the last thirty-six hours.

Separately, her facility started to get a case of the flu going around maybe Thursday last week and spread quickly, infecting a lot of people such that they put the facility in quarantine. Everyone wore masks and gloves, but it left almost as quickly as it came. Saturday night she and I were both good, but she must have contracted it. Just after midnight, going into Sunday, she had vomiting and diarrhea.

They told me about 2:00 in the afternoon that she had a fever and was the only one. I had her sent by ambulance to the hospital where I joined her immediately. It was ok. They put a couple of bags of fluid in her as she was a bit dehydrated. Her fever broke and they gave her anti-nausea and liquid Tylenol for pain. She drank fluids there and ate some crackers,

---

so they sent her off and we returned to the facility around 8:30—past her evening window, but she held on like a trooper.

Monday she was pretty lethargic all day and did not get out of bed. They got her to drink and eat a little.

Tuesday morning was more of the same. Tuesday evening, she was sitting on the edge of her bed, dressed, being fed, and she had a smile on her face. I could not express the joy I was feeling at that moment as I entered her room. I thought, good for you, turning a corner. I was so happy that my eyes welled up. That was 5:00.

I left, and at 8:30 p.m. the nurse called me and said that her red mark on her lower abdomen where she had been rubbing had broken open and generated a wound. They thought she needed to go back to the hospital.

I immediately went back and drove her there myself. After several hours in emergency, they told me very clinically, "There is nothing we can do for her. The tumors are rubbing on the interior of her abdomen making the hole about 3 cm long. She is not strong enough for an operation, and we could not close up the wound even if there were a surgery." Cancer cells do not heal or "stick to each other," as they dumbed it down for me.

They cannot operate, or she will die. They thought it was likely she would die from the wound. They can do nothing for her. There is nothing I can do about it.

It is only a matter of time 'till infection gets inside her and then it is over...she will die.

They sent us home about 1:00 in the morning Wednesday and told me she had "days—maybe a week." Christmas is in a week—her holiday.

I drove her back to the facility and explained the situation to the site RN, Mary. I tucked Maureen in her bed (she had been in her jammies). I kissed her and played a little music for her. We had sway-danced to some music earlier that night before all this. It was hard not to break down in front of her.

I drove home and sobbed the whole way and sobbed alone when I got home. We are now Wednesday morning about 3 a.m.

I changed a pre-scheduled appointment that I had with hospice to, "Now—today!" With a hole there now, I want her to have the best pain meds possible for the best comfort possible. We met at 1:00, and I signed all the forms and met her RN case manager Caitlin, who already knows the facility and staff well.

They will keep her comfortable, the bandage changed, and tend to her needs along with the facility staff and myself. Hospice is for when you are no longer treating to cure—you are treating for comfort and letting things take their course. She cannot be cured. I am losing my baby and it is so hard. I cry and cry.

I called her mom, daughter, son, and best friend Candy last night. Her daughter was just a message to have her call me, as they screen their calls. Her mom did not quite grasp the severity. Her son took it hard. Candy took it the way Candy does—heartfelt but also speaking about how unpredictable life is. That probably is how she copes. It did not help me. My mother called me about a package I had sent. I told her of the situation, and it was twenty questions and a general sorry tone—also did not help.

I went there last night and brought DQ ice cream—vanilla—her favorite. We shared ice cream in her room and listened to Christmas music. A couple of times she wanted to stand. I took the opportunity to sway-dance with her to the music. It took three of us to change her bandage. She was pushing and struggling. It likely hurt. I want the meds to kick in for her pain. I helped her into her pajamas and tucked her in and played more music 'till she could drift off. I kissed her many times and sat there holding her hand.

I am glad that I sent out the Christmas gifts that I did. To her mother, her children, and their spouses, and to each grandchild, I sent gift cards for shoes where a second pair is given to a child in poverty and bracelets that go to fund protection of sea turtles. These were two causes Maureen championed. They will mean something later to people. I hope.

The kids sound like they might be coming up this weekend. Her son will come on Saturday and her daughter on Sunday, maybe. It is always a guess.

I told her son that if he had to drive for UPS, as that happens this time of year, not to worry. He has seen her a few times. He needs to remember her at the good times. He understood but will come anyway.

I love you Maureen.

I always have.

I always will.

It is more than love; it is a deep penetrating warmth in my heart and throughout my body that you provide me. It is happiness, joy, and comfort. I love you taking care of me. Even sick as you are, your hand across my back or kissing me on the top of my head or leaning your head into my hand when I put the backs of my fingers against your cheek—they all comfort me.

There will never be anyone like you again for me. You will never be replaced.

You are beautiful.

You are good and kind.

You are loved by so many.

You are smart.

You are mine for a little while longer.

Please save a spot in heaven for me, as I would really like to see you, and dance with you, again.

Damn work. I will completely clear my schedule the rest of this week. I will think on you constantly.

Thankfully, a short day and then back to you. You are in good hands with the caregivers, and I have told them to call me if you start to slip away. I want to hold your hand as you pass from this place because I do not ever want you to feel abandoned or lonely—only loved.

I cry so much these days and can barely see the keys to type this. I have never sobbed this way. Thank you for that gift too. Kisses and hugs to you always. I love your amazing hugs. I loved rubbing your back last night and helping you into your jammies and tucking you in. It made me feel good, loved, needed, and yours.

Scott's Journal – 12/20/18 (Later the same day)

I was able to be with you in the early afternoon and stay with you for several hours. Your hospice nurse had been in earlier for her first time with you. She changed your bandage and got to know you and gave you some pain meds but was gone when I arrived.

When I entered your room, your jammy bottoms were off, and you were wandering around your room quite lost. Your underwear was soaked and the jammy bottoms slightly damp. The bed sheet slightly damp too. One thing at a time, I thought. Get you cleaned up and then the bed. I took you to the bathroom and found your bandage was gone—red alert. You do not understand not to touch it. That is not your fault.

I quickly flagged down a caregiver to get the med-aid on duty, Tina, and went back to help you remove your underwear and keep you from messing with the wound. I figured it would need to be cleaned and a new dressing applied. Pretty soon I had Tina and two caregivers in there. They changed the bed, and Tina and I got your fresh dressing on. The wound looks a little better—less red and more sort of scabby. I have no hope of it healing. It just looks less ominous.

You were in fresh jammies then but a bit out of sorts with all the running around. You did relax quickly though. With a little soft music, a cookie, and some Fanta, you started to get calm. The hospice Chaplain, Carly, then arrived, and you two met for a few minutes. She got to know you, though you were very quiet, likely still a little agitated by the running around of the rest of us. She liked your Christmas decorations. She asked about us. She asked about our faith.

I told her we got baptized together June 1, 1997 in the Foursquare Church in Eugene. She thought that was rare when a couple can say that. I said we had been dating six months, and you wanted to start fresh, and I wanted to start my life with you. You had been baptized many years prior, but I do not believe I ever had. I mentioned Pastor Ted and the East Hill Church here. I mentioned our short engagement and our promise to Pastor Jerry that we would do marriage counseling after our wedding as there was no time before. I then laughed and explained how we forgot and broke that promise and came clean with Pastor Jerry ten years later when we asked him to renew our vows in our home. He laughed and said that if we were renewing our vows, then we must know what we are doing in respect to marriage.

I told her once Pastor Ted retired, we church shopped for a while. There is a music you like at church and know it when you hear it. I also mentioned occasionally we go to your daughter's Baptist Church when we visit her.

The conversation lagged and she offered to pray over us before she left. She did, and you seemed to hum "Amen". You were present, but not very talkative, which was completely ok.

I stayed with you a while longer but could see your eyes were very heavy. I said I would be back, and you smiled at me as only you can do. I kissed you and hugged you and told you I love you and left.

I returned about 6:30 so I could tuck you in. You beat me and were already asleep in bed. I still sat down and watched you sleep for a while. I played some of your favorite soft music very low, so it soothed rather than woke you. You flinched a few times, woke, adjusted, and slept again. I stroked your arm, your leg, your forehead, all so gently. You just remained in your slumber.

After an hour and many soft songs, I got up to leave and kissed you on your forehead, and you woke a little. You woke with a smile immediately. I love that you do that.

You decided you wanted to roll over and curl up. I kissed you on the temple and said, "Good night pretty lady." You smiled.

I said, "I love you," and you said you loved me too and kept smiling as you drifted off. You at that moment were so content and at peace. I wish all the rest of your days would be like that.

I miss when we slept together for all those years. You would tell me, if I was rolled on my side, to "lie down". That meant I was to lie on my back now and raise my left arm. You then would cuddle in and lie on your right side and on half of me, my arm would come down and around your shoulders. You would say, "It's a thing," and that you had to lie on me for a while before you could go to sleep. You would listen to my breathing and my heart. It brought you peace. You lying on me brought me peace too. Oh, how I miss those nights.

Good night pretty lady. I will see you tomorrow.

As Christmas drew near, Maureen rallied. She stood upright, let people help her dress, ate a little, and continued her pacing, albeit a little shaky. She stayed strong in ways that always amazed me.

Scott's Journal – 12/22/18

The kids came up today. You smiled a little and gave a little hug, but a bit less alert. It could have been the new pain medication. The Dilaudid is fast-acting, but sometimes leaves you a little foggy. We will take the pain relief though. I want you comfortable. You had received a dose twenty minutes before the kids arrived.

The kids met you in the grand room, as the wings were still quarantined from the flu. You spoke a little and smiled a little. I started out with you, but then pulled back to a remote chair to give you more time with just them. It was just your son and daughter and their spouses—no kids. Sadly, when you said nothing, they talked about, and among, themselves: they spoke about UPS or school or whatever—leaving you to fall disengaged.

They do not understand what background noise and isolation does to you. I wish they would receive my coaching. I wish they were more aware. Between them, you saw me sitting remotely. I smiled at you and gave a little wave. You chuckled and gave me a little wave back, which caught all their attention. I love you.

Your daughter got a little teary, so did your son. They walked you around the large room a few times. I let them do so solo, for that one-on-one time. I think your son wanted to be alone with you and did not know when his sister was coming. He walked you to the far side, and you sat together. You spoke, but I do not know what was said. He was having a real hard time with the tears. Your daughter did the same thing, but was not quite as emotional. One time when the two of them walked you around, you came around the corner and looked up at me and said, "That's my husband." I felt such a joy in that. I was thirty feet away and heard it clear as day. They concurred and said yes, that is.

I had to remind you who they all were. You recognized them as safe people, and sometimes that is enough.

Sunday, I brought her mom to the facility, as Maureen had gotten a bit out of sorts on their normal Thursday. Also, I thought adding her to the mix with the kids on Saturday would prove too difficult. Maureen, still weak and a bit out of it, met with her mom. Her mother couldn't help herself and talked about other things that Maureen had no sense of. We restricted the visit to the lobby, so her mom did not catch the flu bug still going around the care facility. I took her mom back to her home and gave her a couple of sentimental gifts intended as from Maureen as likely her last Christmas with her.

AFTD Social Media Post – 12/23/18

KEEPING TOUCH

Merry Christmas and Happy Holidays. It has been over a week since I last posted to this group. I appreciate the support for my off-brand humor as I share things we have learned in our life with FTD. No, reverse that, just our life.

Yesterday, Maureen and I were just sway-dancing as we do. Just the two of us in her room. She stood, the music was playing, so I seized the moment—carpe diem. Our carpes are a little slower these days, but our diems are still EVERY day.

I have read so much on the changes to the senses as the FTD progresses. My wife's eyesight is very narrow, like she is wearing binoculars every day, so I adapt how I approach her and interact with her—stay in front with a little distance. Her hearing is not damaged, but her under-standing of what she hears is, so I speak simply, slowly, and intently as we share. Her tastes and smells are like the hearing, though I have noticed her increased desire for sugar, which is common based on what I have read. My own twenty-year increased desire for sugar is also common and medically described as "no self-control".

However, the sense of touch seems unaffected and remains the best for us. The backrubs continue to be euphoric for her. The hugs, the kisses, the dancing, and the holding hands as we walk or as we just sit, still strongly resonate with her. She is often cold, and my hands are often warm, so I rest the backs of my fingers on her cheek (like feeling for a temperature), and then she leans her head into them. There is something so intimate in that—melting my heart. That instinct, thankfully, is still there.

I love each of these little moments of life. For me, some moments I will find her standing coming up to me while I am sitting (not intending to be a cad—yes, I still stand when a woman comes into the room). I will give her a light hug around the waist, and she leans down and kisses the top of my head—heart aflutter. Fortunately for her, there is far less hair these days on top of my head, so less chance of hair in the mouth.

As I have said before, I cherish these moments of touch as though they are our last. I have not written in a week, as last Tuesday, her inoperable/untreatable cancer tumors bored a hole/wound in her abdomen a little over an inch long. It is not going to heal—it cannot. I have had hospice coming in every day to the memory care facility since to ensure her comfort in what I understand to be her last few days or weeks.

My tears have flown a lot this week: the body tears where your whole body convulses as you sob. You pull it together and keep seeing your loved one, keep touching, keep dancing. To quote another someone we lost too soon, "Nobody puts baby in the corner."

By Christmas Eve, I had called all the critical people in her life to let them know what had happened. I let myself feel encouraged as she rallied because I thought, "Give her a happy Christmas."

On Christmas Eve I saw Maureen early with a soy chai tea latte and ran some errands. I returned by 2:30 to spend the rest of the afternoon and evening with her. She did not eat much the day before and would not touch her dinner now. She got antsy. I asked her if she wanted to go on a drive, and she did. I took her to see the lights at the local raceway (PIR). The racetrack closes for the season, but they decorate the entire area, and cars drive slowly on the track, taking in the wondrous lights. She loved Christmas lights. She thoroughly enjoyed it with a big ol' grin most of the time. However, at the end as we left, she got a little anxious and almost frightened, probably of the dark—something new.

We pulled over in a small lot just before exiting the grounds so she could walk a little. While cold out, the fresh air did her well. The drive home still seemed a bit scary for her. I had to keep reassuring her she had nothing she had to do and that I would take care of her. Guessing, I would say the dark disoriented her. Again, something new. I took her home rather than trying to add the lights at Peacock Lane.

She calmed down as I spoke to her and we got off the freeway, so we stopped for a burger and fries and milkshake to try and get some calories in her. She ate half of each back in the grand room. She immediately calmed down.

I got her into her jammies without incident, and we lay down together and listened to several bits of Christmas music as she drifted off. She liked having me lie there with her. I had the lights of her tree turned on. She studied them and smiled. She seemed happy and content.

"Did you like the lights tonight?" I asked.

"Yeah," she replied, apparently now over the fears of the dark.

I got up and kissed her and said, "Merry Christmas Maureen."

"Merry Christmas," she answered as her lids got heavy.

"I love you baby."

"I love love love you," she replied.

"I'll be back in the morning," I finished. She drifted off.

Christmas morning, I woke up alone in our old house. I had put up no decorations there or anything to remind me of the season and had done all the decorating just at her place. I quickly dressed and went to the facility so she would wake up with me Christmas morning. However, I knew she would surely wake up like just any other day. I hate that FTD robbed her of that—her favorite holiday.

We ate together that morning and evening. I had brought her a couple gifts. She no longer understood how to unwrap, so I just placed them in gift bags. Even that confounded her: she looked at the bags, not reasoning they contained presents inside. We opened them together. One had a small silk poinsettia for her room. She liked it. Fortunately, she understood and smelled it. I had bought some scent and sprayed it previously, so she made the connection. I got her pajamas and a small album with pictures of her kids and grandkids. We went simple—no reason to complicate things.

Later that day, I decluttered her room a bit. I left one of the snow globes and most of the snowmen. I would do more over the subsequent days—a little at a time, so as not to overwhelm her with change. I had no idea how much time I had left with her.

The weekend after Christmas, I brought Maureen her chai. She started happy to see me, yet in fifteen minutes went to telling me to leave and pushing my hand away from holding hers three different times. I did not understand the trigger that I had hit, assuming that I even hit a trigger. FTD can act randomly like that. Not worried, I knew it would pass but respected her wishes and left her to drink her chai.

She had acted more upset, bothered, or lightly angry each morning since Christmas Day. However, when I came later those nights to tuck her in, she seemed much more relaxed and receptive. One night that week she needed to scoot in her bed to lie down but could not figure how to do it. I cradled and picked her up to move her and said, "This is just like when I carried you across the door on our wedding day."

She smiled and said, "You are are...best baby ever."

The next night as she lay in bed, she told me, "I love you so so much."

The moods would come and go, and I rolled with them. I savored the sweetest moments and gave her space in the harder ones. I kept thinking since December 18th and the hole in her side that "this was it," but she rallied and, while weak, stayed with us.

She still ate very little, so we tried to give her more smaller meals throughout the day to make up for it. She still drank her Ensure. I brought chicken nuggets, and she liked those, but not every time. We mixed in snacks. With medicines we had hits and misses with her wanting to take them and then not. If she resisted, I would take a break and put them down and ask again five minutes later, which tended to have better success.

I caught myself thinking about what her last moments would feel like a lot—and always "the when". I had no interest in hastening her passing, but I also did not want her to suffer. Would she feel pain at the end? Well, I thought, hospice would keep that from happening. Would she pass in her sleep in the middle of the night? Would she feel alone or abandoned? Would fortune allow me to sit with her at the moment she passed and hold her hand and make her feel loved, treasured, comforted? I had a lot of uncertainty and tears.

I had a hard time getting into the holiday spirit myself and trying to keep her in it too. I still played music as we slowly walked. I still tried to integrate a little spin or a slow sway-dance in our time at least once a day. I still tried to show my love and caring for her. I did my best, but I could not shake the feeling that I had not done enough.

I also wrongly started pushing away people. Maureen had not yet died, but I still actively grieved, and not in a healthy way. I no longer went to the gym, nor did I eat or sleep well.

My mother called with the pat, "Let me know if there is anything I can do." She caught me in a bad mood. I snapped at her but also released just a little of the last thirty-plus years of frustration.

"What are you offering to do? Honestly, what is that offer? You have known for two and a half years that Maureen has dementia but have not come down to visit once. Have I gone up? No. I am caring for her. But if you are offering to do "anything you can," then why not come see your daughter-in-law before she is on her death-bed? I mean, have you done "anything" in thirty-plus years? I took care of my first car, my college, my homes, my jobs, my moves, my wedding, my trips, my career, and now my wife's health. Not you. You have done plenty of those things for my brother and sister. I did not grant you grandchildren, so you really did not have the time for me—is that it? My most vivid childhood memory of Dad is him holding me by my neck 'till my feet dangled off the floor with a look of bloodlust in his face like he could just snap my neck. This was spurred on by you crying over a minor disagreement. I did not insult you, just disagreed. However, any child expressing their own opinion in our house would throw Dad into a rage. Do you know I nearly ran away twice? Once I made it out the window, on a bus, and downtown in the middle of the night just to turn around and come back. I thought I'd be damned if I let them rob me of my childhood. My family taught me nothing. Everything in my life from relationships, to work, to finance, to communication, to everything has been from self-reliance. I was never good enough for you two, so I thought I might as well rely on myself to figure it out. And you know what? I did just fine on my own."

I paused, knowing I had crossed a line but selfish enough to not care. While not a good excuse, my grief proved a powerful catalyst.

After a bit of silence, I could hear my mother say, "We did support you. We did praise you."

Because I had already behaved like a prick, I fired back, "That is horseshit. I can think of countless times where I would sit down with you guys to try and share an accomplishment of mine, and the first things out of your mouths were not 'good job' but rather what my brother, my sister, my brother-in-law, or my father was doing that was bigger and grander and of more importance. Always comparing. It has gotten so I don't bother sharing with you anymore—what is the point? No support when I ran for Mayor. No support when I became a Principal in my company—an international design firm for God's sake. In fact, I remember when I told you two. The first words out of Dad's mouth were, "So how many people are in the firm?" I told him it was about twelve hundred. He said, "Oh is that all? It is much smaller than I thought. Boeing has tens of thousands." I remember thinking he was an ass, and all that I did meant nothing to you. Well, you know who it DID mean something to? The woman lying in a care facility dying right now—my beautiful wife and your daughter-in-law."

While not at all my normal self, I also could not deny that I said those awful things that had built up over the years and just exploded out. My mother said a quiet goodbye, and I hung up. Weeks later, I apologized, though she had already forgiven me in some way as moms do. I work to make amends still.

Caregivers need to remember, we will have human moments, and we will all do things we will immediately, or later, regret. We all have weaknesses where we just do not show the strength that we want for ourselves. We will push people away. We have to take the time to reset, apologize, reconnect, and soldier on. Some further self-care tips:

1. Forgive yourself.

2. Get a massage if that is your thing.

3. Pray or seek spiritual counsel—again, if that is your thing.

4. Read a book on grief. I recommend Megan Devine's *It's OK that you're not OK.*

New Year's Eve came and Maureen felt pretty good—thirteen days since the appearance of the hole in her abdomen. I had asked the med-aid, Tina, to speak to hospice about changing the timing of her anti-depressant (Mirtazapine) to the middle of the day instead of the evening to space it off a bit from her evening pain med (a minimum dosage of Dilaudid). This kept her mood stabilized through more of the day rather than her having minor crashes mid-afternoon.

I stayed with Maureen 'till 8:30 that night, leaving her lying in bed and near asleep. I had played her music. She swayed with me: in the chair with just her arms around me and also a bit while standing. I brought her Dairy Queen, and she ate some and enjoyed it. She told me she loved me "so so much." What more could I ask for, given all that went on inside her body and mind?

I heard fireworks going off as I journaled—maybe because it had just turned midnight in New York. I could not get into much of the festivity alone back in the old house without my baby with me. Normally, on New Year's Eve, we would dance at some venue, including a couple of times on a boat—such great memories. We would dance the night away and watch the sky light up with fire-works, sometimes just at home from our floating gazebo. I loved our time together so much—loved her so much.

January came and went with its ups and downs, but she perse-vered. She kept outliving the doctor's predictions. It blessed me with some more time with her. Maureen had always lived strong.

Spacing out the meds seemed to really help her mood. It brought her back to just the language side of the FTD and put the crashes at bay. For all I know though, the disease might have also just naturally progressed in that way. I do not think she had to consciously fight it off, although she always looked weary. The physical toll seemed obvious most days.

We still walked a lot, held hands a lot, and ate together daily. I would take her out on short one-hour trips for her chai or a milkshake and stop at a park and people watch from the car. She would smile, not say much, and then get antsy to walk. We would try walking outside, but she simply got too cold (no matter the layers). I took her back to the facility, where we would walk the halls repeatedly.

I left some of the Christmas decorations up 'till late in the month, slowly removing them and making it last. Taking out the tree made it feel barren, so I brought in a small end table that she and I had stained together several years prior. She saw it, and I asked her if she remembered us staining it together. She said yes. Sometimes I wondered if she just gave affirmative answers out of habit or if she really remembered. We enjoyed doing projects together throughout our marriage.

Her eating remained moody. She did not want to eat some meals at all and finished others. I honestly think it just came down to when she got hungry but did not know how to express it—she was never a three-meal-a-day kind of gal. She grazed on the snacks I brought. Sometimes I brought fruits and veggies and cheese and other healthy things. Sometimes I just focused on the calorie-dense foods. She still liked her cookies and her Fanta.

For much of January, the place remained quarantined for the flu. Residents were separated into two smaller wings and got isolated to their units if they showed symptoms. They required visitors to wear masks and gloves—a small price to pay to see my dear wife.

They closed the grand room. Maureen and I cheated a couple of nights and snuck out to sit there and listen to her music. After she started to get sleepy, I brought her back to her room. She told me, "You you...you best for me." Those things melted my heart. I fought back the tears and told her, "You're the best for me too." We held hands as she drifted off.

While I cherished those moments, we had many unpleasant days too—in fact, most days. However, I could still mine one or two good moments out of even those. I also cried a lot.

Some of it I did to myself. When I took down her Christmas things, I removed her Christmas sweaters. I washed them and heard them tumbling in the dryer. I thought likely she would never see them or wear them again. I cried. I folded them nicely and put them away for the season. They reminded me of our winter morning walks on a sunny yet brisk and cold day. I remembered that crispness in the air and the smell of fireplaces coming alive. We would return to the comfort of our warm home and lie on the couch snuggled under a blanket—fresh, soothing, and enveloping me. I treasured those good memories, but they still made me cry.

Some nights I had it bad, and I almost broke down by her bedside. She would go on about things, "Just just not...right." She had a hard time finding her words, but I could see the sadness, anger, or simply her frustrated confusion at the state of her world in her eyes and tone of voice.

I felt so bad. I teared up and apologized to her that I could not make things better but that I tried. Sometimes, something in her mind would shift in those moments. With my head dropped down on her bed and tears on my cheeks, she once placed her hand behind my head and said, "Ok. He is ok...come." I looked up and she scooted over in this little twin bed and kept repeating, "Come with, with, with...her."

I got out of the chair and lay on the bed next to her as best I could, my face cuddled on her shoulder. She bent her arm and used her hand to cradle my cheek and said, "I love love...you so so so much. You my best baby." We still took care of each other.

I sympathized with her agitation. They started having her sleep in a zipped onesie to keep her from messing with her wound at night. With FTD, she simply did not understand to leave the bandage alone. I suppose it felt like something to explore or something in the wrong place. It did not feel right and set her off as something out of sorts. That, combined with an in and out status of flu quarantine, simply stressed her with the changing routines.

In that agitation, she stopped even drinking the Ensure, or would dump it. I went to Starbucks and bought ten of the white, reusable, lightweight, plastic cups with slotted lids. I labelled them all (lids and cups) with her name. From that point on, staff and I would put her Ensure in those cups, and she drank them happily.

Sometimes we lucked out and timed a weekly visit from her mother for "coffee", where Maureen would manage a great mood. They would talk: Maureen not making sense of course but laughing and getting us all laughing—good times. I would take her mother home, and she would comment that Maureen's dementia had subsided and was perhaps getting better. I would simply state, "She had a good day." I would then let it go. I had given up explaining that Maureen would never get better, that the tumors could breach her stomach at any time, and then we would have just hours or days 'till the end. I thought it was best to let her have the good memories and cope as she needed to.

I let myself get in a dark mood sometimes. I felt like FTD had robbed us of the rest of our lives together. At the same time, the everyday question of "Will today be the day I lose my baby?" still persisted. I did not want to lose her. I sobbed at the idea of losing her. I also feared that the moment, the exact moment, that I let my guard down, God would take her.

I lectured myself daily to let go of the dread and celebrate the magnificence of the ordinary—the magical moments. I could not easily see them, find them, or make them. After all, Maureen did seem like she got a second wind by the end of the month. She got out of bed on her own, continued her pacing, and showed increased curiosity. I just went with it and supported her any way I could.

AFTD Social Media Post – 1/28/19

SHOES

"I've worn lots of shoes. I bet if I think about it real hard, I can remember my first pair of shoes. Mama said they'd take me anywhere." For Forrest Gump, his shoes took him all over the world. For my wife, her shoes often took her out to go get more shoes: racks and racks, shelves and shelves, boxes and boxes of shoes. I would find myself apologizing to my wife for taking over the closet with my two shirts, one pair of pants, and some old sneakers.

Nowadays, in her memory care facility, she is down to four pairs plus slippers. However, I will often find that she is wearing only one shoe. No worries. I just shout "Hi baby!" with my arms swung wide. She sees me and smiles. We walk slowly together and hug. I just tell her I love her and tell her how pretty she looks. I wait 'till we walk a few steps and then ask, "Are you walking like a pirate?"

"What?!" she asks.

I say, "Somebody took your other shoe." I never say, "You lost your shoe." That puts it on her and makes her feel stupid. She looks down and says, "Yeah."

Now I will often notice that the remaining one is on the wrong foot too, which cannot be comfortable. I will sit her down on the nearest bench and suggest we remove this shoe and go find the other one together. She is then in socks. If she seems at all uneasy, I take my shoes off too and say, "Let's go look for shoes together." Off we go holding hands. My wife shuffles now and looks down a lot, so without me, stubbing her toe can easily happen. Hence, I try to keep her shoes on and because I like to use "hence".

Pretty soon we find the stray near a chair in the hall or on an end table next to an abandoned Starbucks reusable cup that she finished her Ensure from. I collect her "donations" around the facility as we walk, but I say nothing about it to her.

I then ask her to sit, and I rub her toes a little and then put on her shoes. While on my old decrepit knees, I look up at her and hold both hands and ask her if that feels good. Sometimes I get a yes, and sometimes I get a story void of nouns, "I think they did it a while ago, and it wasn't good."

"It sounds like it wasn't good," I respond.

"Exactly," she replies. We continue to walk.

I know we are blessed that she can still walk and talk and recognize me. She cannot recall my name without a prompt but remembers I am her husband about 70% of the time. She always remembers that I am a safe person and that I love her, but maybe thinks sometimes we are just dating. "I don't care. It was like olden times. We was like peas and carrots again. Every week I put pretty flowers in her room." – Paraphrasing Forrest. After all. I DO put flowers in her room every week.

So far, I have had another six weeks with her since her December 18th diagnosis with a cancer-caused hole in her side and "days or weeks" to live. Since then, we got one more Christmas, one more New Year's, and countless more tender moments together among the challenges. She got shingles last week. Apparently, her body was bored and thought, "Let's spice things up a bit."

We take it together every step. I am making the most of this time—good and bad. I am prepared for the day she passes. By prepared, I mean prepared to be devastated and bawl uncontrollably—you know, prepared. Per Gump, "Life is a box of chocolates. You never know what you're gonna get."

Yes, shingles. FTD, cancer, and now...shingles. WTH?!?!

I got the surprise while I rubbed her back under her sweater and felt bumps. It shocked me that others had known about this and said nothing to me. Staff had noticed them two to three days prior but had put lotion on them. They did not think to tell me or the med-aid. Sometimes the ball still gets dropped in a care facility with good people. I insisted a real nurse see her who confirmed in five seconds—yes, shingles. She got on meds five times a day, but she had to continue to endure the onesies 'till they cleared up. It healed quickly, but my poor darling.

Post holidays, she received a few more visitors, but even good people tend to disappear at these times. They just do not know how to react or what to do. That behavior comes more from our grief culture than the individuals.

A cousin of hers, Margo from Georgia, came to town and stopped by briefly. Her mother had died with Alzheimer's years earlier and had some knowledge of a person's decline with dementia. I explained the differences to her. One of Maureen's nephews came to visit as well. We shared some laughter, but pain too at seeing her so frail.

Maureen had some pain, but not often. Hospice kept it well managed. Hospice saw her most days. When I started them December 19, 2018 (the day after her hole appeared), I understood that no longer would we try to treat or cure, but rather just aim to give her comfort. I did not know the wisdom of that choice that so many before me had made. I will not know the rest of my life.

We continued to have tender moments. Some I jotted down, just a word or phrase I found endearing, and others I just sat and treasured the moment—not trying to capture or record. I think about how people, and me on occasion, are always so anxious to whip out their phones and take a picture or video rather than simply sitting back and taking in the moment.

I did capture a few evening moments on video though. I play them back still, just to hear her voice.

I liked the quiet evenings when the two of us just talked softly in her room. We held hands. She lay in her bed drifting off. I played her music. We exchanged endearments. She seemed content.

I also liked many of our middays. She would stroll back and forth, sometimes talkative with plenty on her mind, convinced she was telling me a story. It did not matter that she said just a jumble of words. I liked her word salad and would repeat a couple of words back to her, giving her affirmation and launching her into more with perhaps a bit of laughter or animation.

I even occasionally liked the dark times when, unhappy with me for some imagined situation, she would chastise me. Sometimes I could walk with her and hold her hand and eventually turn her around. Sometimes I left for an hour and let it pass and came back. She would start anew, happy to see me again, and would greet me as someone long lost and dear to her.

I loved that she remembered me as someone important, safe, and loving. I think for the most part she remembered our times together and as a married couple, but even if she did not and just loved me, I could live with that too.

Some nights when I tucked her in and played her music, she reached out and pulled me close. She would place her hand behind my head and pat it while humming along to the songs and say, "love those." She would then bring my fingers to her lips and kiss them. All this to soothe me, who she instinctively saw in front of her as so very broken.

What we had remained so very special. SHE remained so very special.

I kept reading up on Maureen's condition and things to try and came across a list of six Beatles songs that neurologist claimed to have positive effects on people with autism and some other forms of mental agitation. I downloaded them and created a second playlist for Maureen, as she already liked the Beatles from her childhood. On one particularly agitated afternoon, I played that list, and she hummed or sang to each of the tunes. She seemed very calm. I do not know if these songs had that particular effect or not, but I tried to provide that sort of specific care for her. I tried to read and adapt and apply and adjust. I would try, in moderation, various foods, sounds, smells, and activities. I wanted her happy and comfortable. I could not get her healthy, so I tried for everything else.

I still of course played her standby list. We walked slowly. We sat quietly. We listened to her music. She often hummed and seemed to find some peace at many points. One night, about three songs in, she said, "I love those songs." I smiled and said I know—a tear rolling down my cheek. She had become so innocent in so many ways. Simple things brought her joy that escape the rest of us so often.

In those moments, we would sit, and I would kiss her hand as I often did. That month, out of the blue, she picked up my hand and kissed the back of it. I thanked her and teared up. She had not done that for over a year.

I would walk and talk to her and my voice would sometimes crack remembering easier times. She once stopped in that care facility, so frail, and looked at me (she did not do that typically, as, at that point, she hung her head almost always), and she hugged me around the neck and said, "You love her." I knew what she meant regardless of the pronouns. I said, "Yes I do," and hugged her back.

I exchanged Maureen's January decorations with Valentine's ones. Pinks and reds surrounded her, and she liked those colors. I went with more pink than red to keep it calmer. I hung a twenty-year-old Valentine's collage I made for her way back on our first Valentine's Day after we married. She had liked it and kept it hung in the house. It included phrases and thoughts from early on in our dating. It also had vintage Valentine's cards posted in it.

The same old house I had moved back into for five months now had received a couple of nibbles here and there, but no offers yet. I kept my footprint in it small and always cleaned when I left each day to keep it pristine for unannounced buyer walks that might creep up. Most onlookers simply could not get past the steep driveway, and I could do nothing about that. Our savings rapidly diminished to near nothing by that point.

While I still worked, I also withdrew from a lot of people: messages, texts, e-mails, phone calls, social media—I pulled back from most of that. I worked, and I stayed with her.

I still remained connected with the online AFTD support group. They published one of my stories in their e-newsletter. While I found that nice, I did not want to celebrate me. I wanted to let everybody know what a wonderful person Maureen remained in the midst of the FTD. I wanted to share what a strong and courageous and good soul she had.

But I also found it a place to support others. I tried to do that at least as often as I posted myself. So many people struggle with FTD, either themselves or for their loved ones: parents, spouses, kids, extended family, and friends. With our mutual sharing, we taught each other, comforted each other, inspired each other.

Caregiving can prove daunting and wear you down. I remember reading one post where the gentlemen's mother had developed FTD, and he felt he simply did not have the strength to do the caregiving. I told him, "Strength is the coat we wrap others with, leaving ourselves to shiver in the cold. We are left with grace that will warm us from the inside without us knowing it."

I thought about giving someone your strength so they can live strong in adversity. That seemed to me like one of the most graceful acts a person can perform for another. Selflessness leaves us vulnerable. I thought about how Maureen and I had lived our marriage and how we each had done that for the other. We always had complete trust—even in our worst times.

I still kept trying outings, just to stimulate her mind. I saw her cut flowers in her room dying, reminding me that week I had forgotten to bring her fresh ones. I also knew she had not ventured out in over a week. Cold and foggy that morning, I still asked her if she wanted to go on a drive, and she did. We went to a nearby grocery store and got the flowers. I had her help pick out the bouquet best she could. We stopped by a drive-through as well for chai and a croissant. I got her back before lunch and arranged her flowers and broke apart her croissant for her—small victories.

Midday, she often explored. She would sometimes walk through people's conversations. She would hear words of their conversations and think she had to reply in some fashion with her head still hung or a slight glance upward. Sometimes others pleasantly accepted this, but other times it was met with a rebuke from a fellow resident. Understandably, not all remain tolerant. I asked caregivers to watch those incidents and try to help her navigate out of them. For all I knew, she thought she still lived at home and she needed to mingle with these "guests".

Conversely, she did not at all want to be around the games they played. Other residents played this game with foam paddles and a big balloon or beach ball. They would hit it back and forth. Maureen did not like that game and did not play it. I think something like that must have put her too much on edge. She could no longer make those quick types of decisions.

In the evenings, we would walk and play her music, and often we danced. I placed Springsteen's "Secret Garden" on her playlist. Once, while we danced, she stopped and slowly and deliberately took the lapels of my jacket and kissed my chest and said she loved me. On another occasion, while walking and having a hard time fighting back some tears, she caught sight of my face and saw me sad with wet eyes. She looked me dead in the eyes and said, "I love you." I told her thank you and that I loved her too. A couple of times a month she would have those lucid moments, and I wanted to hold onto them. Those moments, while brief, will stay with me always.

By early February, the shingles had healed completely, and they let her return to her preferred and recognizable clothes. She slept better in her soft and familiar pajamas. She really did not like those onesies.

I appreciated that shift because some staff would dress her in just a onesie in the middle of the day. No other resident dressed like that. Everyone else wore their normal clothes. The little things like dignity still needed to matter. I told them to place a sweater over her when they put her in the onesie so it would look like a top and pants. I asked them to always think about dignity and what they would want for themselves. The rare caregiver would put themself in Maureen's shoes. The long-timers did. The new ones kind of just "showed up".

She rarely had any more outbursts or agitated behavior, but she had also grown a bit quiet. She would stare off more and utter fewer words. Occasionally, I could get a jovial conversation going, but far more seldom. I confirmed her meds had stayed at the minimum dosages. Pain control seemed good, but I did not want her drugged into a non-verbal state. With FTD though, that communication piece can become more non-verbal. I made sure I continued to support her confidence.

I still took her to see her mom once a week, but the February visits had turned out poorly. Maureen typically looked right through her mom. Her mom of course cried, as she saw herself losing her daughter. While she had watched that happening for a while now, it finally hit home. Maureen never got much out of these visits anymore in her mother's apartment with nothing familiar. I proposed that we change to me picking her up and taking her to Maureen, and that maybe she would be more responsive in a familiar day-to-day environment. She agreed to this. I knew that if Maureen could communicate it, she would want these visits to continue, so I kept doing them, almost every Thursday morning.

In truth, most visits after that did not go well. I brought her mother to see her every week through the spring and summer, but Maureen remained typically dismissive of it, and that certainly hurt her mother. She wanted Maureen to recognize her, but they did not have the closeness that her mother wanted now. Her mother had waited too long.

Dementia often brings out the real person without the filters. While Maureen certainly loved her mother and had always acted very kind and attentive with her before, she felt no real closeness now. She no longer had a filter telling her to show affection if she did not feel it. Maureen saw just a woman now, which she only sometimes recognized—not so much a close friend to get chatty with. Maureen treated her somewhat platonically now, as she knew no better. As I said, sometimes Maureen looked right through her.

Sadly, the staff continued to let Maureen roam the halls at night. The multiple sit-downs with administration and staff and my written direction should have taken care of it. Unfortunately, staff changes rarely included briefings about residents, so I would find myself constantly retraining new staff. Four out of seven nights, I would tuck Maureen in. A couple of nights, I would have dinner with her and let staff tuck her in, so she would allow others to do it. I would tell staff, "Remember, she needs to be in bed by 8:00, starting to dress for bed by 7:30." Sure enough, I would call at about 8:30 to confirm they got Maureen in bed, and at least once a week, they did not. I would drive back and find her wandering the halls, or in response to my call, they had just changed her and put her in bed. New caregivers complained that Maureen put up a struggle and once had "pulled on her finger."

I explained, "You cannot put Maureen in bed late or she gets cranky and fights receiving care. Her mental defenses falter, and she does not know better. This is on her write-up sheet. You can't blame her."

I would sit and apologize to Maureen for them. She would lie there visibly agitated and pull her covers up to her chin, "They... just..."

"I know baby. They mess with you."

"Yeah, mess," she would reply.

"They are trying to help you with your pajamas. Do you like your pajamas? They're soft," I would redirect.

"Yeah," she would trail off. She would stroke her pajamas and seemed to contemplate that idea of "soft". That had always appealed to her. We would enter a department store and even if we had no intention of buying clothes, she would feel the fabrics of sweaters and tops as we walked by. The feel determined whether she would look further. After softness came the neckline: rounded or only a slight V—nothing plunging. She typically gravitated to long sleeves and no exposed midriff. She remained modest her whole life. Even now in this room with her mind ravaged by the disease, she stroked the sleeve to feel the softness.

I needed to give her the time and environment to relax. I would turn on the CD player in her room with some of her favorite discs. The staff started using the player in the mornings, so her mood stayed happy and light as they dressed her. At night, I would stroke her arm or hold her hand lightly for a few songs. Sometimes she would hum, and sometimes just drift off after quite a bit of time. Sometimes it took ten minutes, sometimes more than an hour. FTD makes your mind race, and late at night it often took a while to undo that.

Bless you my baby. Tomorrow is a new day.

Monsters and Poppies

I knock on your heart's door.
The monster darkens your room, and howls echo from
all directions
Disorienting your senses.
You can't locate my knock.

The monster sleeps for a moment, so I
Steal away inside with you.
"I love you." "I love you too."
"I love having you as my wife." "Yeah..."

The monster wakes and roars, "He does that, did that, and
I saw it there."
Shut out again. The monster barring the door.
Memories sifting through her mental walls are just mist.
Brain fog they call it aptly.

Humor scarcely surfaces, yet loving
Endures its weary flight knowing
Purpose will carry its wings and form poetry
Savored as winter tea.

Dozens of tulip bulbs primed to bloom but kept dormant
Beneath the surface by the creature's cold breath and
viny reach
Choking out life save for the stray outlier it snorts and
muses,
"I will squash that one soon enough."

You are my dream river flowing gently yet
Whipped by the wicked wind into that mist
Crashing against the stones
Not of our own hands

Our moment but an ember cupped in our laced
Hands from that wicked wind. Fragile and turning to dust
Leaving my hands empty, wanting
Your fingers again intertwined.

No poppies yet offered to you.
I will still insist on Cala lilies.
Chasing your breath that
Moves this world.

AFTD Social Media Post – 2/14/19

VALENTINE'S DAY

"You had me at hello." – Jerry Maguire

As a hopeless romantic, Valentine's Day is a big deal for me. I love spoiling my wife. We used to go every Valentine's Day to a steakhouse here called Ringside—never a bad meal in twenty years. We would also go there for our birthdays and anniversary and would squeeze in another excuse, like Flag Day. When I proposed to Maureen, we celebrated that same evening at Ringside (if she said 'no', it might have been a drive-through).

As many have noted, FTD forces us to change our traditions. I have also learned that we cannot create new traditions. What she could manage two years ago, she could not do last year, and even less so this year. I still make plans for her, but I also prepare for it to all go to hell—no fault of hers, just FTD.

For her peace of mind, I spread it out. Last Sunday, I painted her nails. The FTD makes her fidget, so I cannot find a manicurist with the patience. Counting last Sunday, I have painted nails...once. I have seen it done, I thought. If you can become a master painter by watching Bob Ross, I can certainly paint some nails. I bought what I needed, picked the best time of the day, brought her an easy lunch and drink, and took our time. Sadly, I forgot my reading glasses, which would have made it sooooo much easier. They did not turn out half bad. She was a trooper to keep so still. I was blowing on her nails for all I was worth to get them dry before she moved. I got lucky...and lightheaded (later I was told they make a product for fast drying).

I brought her roses, a card, and a small box of chocolates. I just sat them in her room early in the day without making a big deal. I wanted to minimize the stimuli. She found them on her own later. So far so good.

I asked her a few days prior if she wanted to wear a dress. She said yes. I reminded her for a few days, so it would not be a surprise. I brought one of her favorites—super easy to put on. Uh...no! She fought it, so I stopped immediately and just lay it on the bed. We walked for a while and later went back to her room. She said, "That's MY dress." "Yes, I brought it for you." "Well, thank you," she said. It became her idea and much better.

That was 2:00. Her facility was hosting a Valentine's dinner at 4:00. They had name placards for your reserved table, flowers, etc. There was even a harpist that my wife hummed along to. The spacing of two hours was to make sure she was relaxed. There was going to be more people and more noise than normal. It started out ok, but she got cold, so I rushed a coat on her. We slow danced a little to the harp music, but then she wanted to walk. They brought dinner in three courses. My wife has trouble focusing on one dish. I could start to see her unravel and walked her more. We walked in a circle, and each time we passed our table, I took a bit of food and put it in her mouth. She chewed and walked. Soon I took her to the quiet of her room.

This was not a traditional candlelit evening, but we made it the best we could. I am not sure we will get another Valentine's Day, so I relaxed and lowered my expectations and let her lead this dance.

"So, it's not gonna be easy. It's gonna be really hard. We're gonna have to work at this every day, but I want to do that because I want you. I want all of you. Forever. You and me... every day." – The Notebook

---

Despite the challenges, some days, her FTD just faded into the background like something that you could almost forget.

Scott's Journal – 2/18/19

Today was a good day.

I brought Maureen her soy chai and some pastries, and I decided to splurge and get me a drink too. I came to her room, and she was there, up and dressed, and smiling and in a good mood. We sat together in her room and drank and ate and talked. She was in good spirits with a little laughter, lots of smiles, and lots of love. It reminded me of our lazy Sunday mornings, just the two of us, where we did the same.

I played different music, some harp music she had heard before. It was so pleasant, just magical, as though we had been transported back in time before all this FTD and cancer and just the two of us with our whole lives ahead of us.

I did not want it to end. We walked some and had a good time.

I left her at lunch with her seated at a table and told her I would be back. She kissed me and said that was fine, with a smile.

I came back about 4 o'clock and, after a bit, helped her with her dinner. She ate a little but not too much. We walked and talked a bit more—still in good spirits. She teased me a bit. The actual words were not understandable, but she would say something and I would try to respond, and then that little wry smile would come up, and she said she was kidding. She was messing with me. She loves and trusts me that much. She knows me and delights in me being there.

I left after dinner but could not help myself and returned about 7:30. She was in bed and resting, but her eyes were still open. I played a couple of quiet songs and watched her fall asleep. I gently rubbed her hand and leg and just enjoyed being with her.

Though I believe they managed her pain well, her whole physical stature definitely had changed in the last year. I believe she weighed in the low nineties at this point.

She mostly shuffled now and hung her head low. I would hug her, and she would keep her head bowed and sort of bury her forehead into my chest. When I kissed her, she would kiss my shirt at my chest level—still affectionate but definitely weary. I feared it all had just beaten her down slowly.

In the mornings, she stayed a bit more alert and would sort of look up through the tops of her eyes and see me and smile. She got more talkative and animated. One morning visit, I said, "I have to go back to work, but I will come back right afterward." She looked at me and smiled and said, "He always comes back to me." It felt good that she had that level of comfort.

Some afternoons, I would come in and look for her and would find her in the small chapel. I did not know if she picked up on the religious tones or if she just sought a quiet place. I asked her if she liked this church, but she never answered. I knew she had a hard time finding her own room.

By late-afternoon and in the evening though, she would just get very sedate. I had noticed that around 6 p.m. (getting earlier and earlier) she would get flush in the face and start obsessively rearranging things in her room, very disoriented. She could see and not see at the same time—lost in a fog.

As we walked the halls, she would occasionally say, "This, this place...is, is, is just...nice." That certainly relieved my heart.

I would ask, "Are the people ok?"

She would reply, "Yes, yes people...are, are, we are nice." That also made me feel good.

She did still sometimes get bothered by them when they changed her or showered her, as she did not like being messed with and remained fiercely modest. Yet her agitation lasted only briefly now, and she would immediately get back to herself. It had become routine.

Chapter 11

Rallying Again

*I*n many ways, I think that to Maureen routine had broken down to simply coping. They would get her up, get her dressed, get her to breakfast, help her, sit her in the grand room or at the TV or back to her room, check on her, talk to her, get her to lunch, get her to the grand room, get her to her room get her back out for dinner, get her to the TV, get her to her room, get her in her pajamas, and lay her down. They simply did not know how to engage her and left that to me. Sometimes though, she would change things up herself.

Maureen would wander the halls, and they would lose track of her and go find her. On occasion, if a resident left a door open, she would wander into their room and sit there. They would lose her and search for her.

If one of her favorite med-aids worked "the cart", she would walk and talk to them and just have a long chat as they made out the medications for each of the residents. She would just talk pleasantly and ask questions and make conversation, but with her word salad, they simply did not respond other than to give her pleasant platitudes back, so she felt welcome. She would then walk off and wander to a comfortable or familiar chair and sit when she got tired.

She did not reach out to make any chit-chat with other residents, as she had lost so much ability to initiate. Some residents did approach her. Some residents would grab her hand and lead her around, and sometimes she went along, and other times she became agitated and pulled away. They would persist. When I came in, I would watch from a distance and then intervene if she seemed tired or agitated.

I would give her one of my "Ta-Das" and "save her" from the situation. We would sit down, and I would ask her if she felt good. She'd reply, "No, no, no, they, they, they...just...don't."

"Did you walk with one of the ladies?"

"Yeah...but, but, but, but...they just don't."

It felt contrary for her. Her body language conveyed a very bothered state of mind and heart. I had to rely on this, as she had difficulty expressing it with speech—especially when under duress. I understood. She would then take my hand in her hand and just keep patting it, then run her hand up and down mine. I would watch the agitation just melt away without me saying anything. With me, she took control back.

She simply found it hard to initiate a conversation or communicate her feelings or say "no". I tried to act as her voice and asked the caregivers to watch in case Maureen let herself get bullied. I understood the residents never intentionally bullied, but when they made Maureen go a certain way or do a certain thing, whether she could voice it or not, it inadvertently became bullying. I asked the staff to also, like me, act on her behalf.

I had ongoing struggles with staffing—not any individual in particular. I would train them up, and most of it would take. I tried to make sure, due to childhood trauma, that she did not have a male caregiver change her. It happened a couple of times due to a shortage of staff, and she really fought it. I begged them, "PLEASE READ THE FILE." I painstakingly included all of these guides, but inevitably, turnover in those positions often created "fires" to put out. I did reorientation every other week with someone new.

I would see minor physical things like a right cheek suddenly puffy. I brought it up to the med-aid, who seemed to only notice when I brought it up. She took a picture and sent it to hospice. They called me and suggested a little fluid had collected and should pass in a couple days. It did, but it seemed odd that only I noticed these kinds of issues. While this felt unfair to Maureen and the other residents, it remains a broken piece of the industry.

Maureen received visitors very seldomly at this point, often unannounced or vague—"sometime this weekend." This required my outings with her to stay nimble. I'd have to adjust for these visitors, as I knew it was important too.

She still saw her mother weekly, but Maureen had a hard time sitting for long. She wanted to walk, and her mother's bad knees would prevent her from doing so. She would sit 'till I could circle Maureen back. I never did figure out the right formula for her mother's visits so that both of them would get something out of it. I do not think a formula existed.

FTD has no right recipe. Moods frequently change. Even with our own interactions, sometimes they would hit and sometimes miss. Focusing on the calories, I would bring her a chicken sandwich, fries, and a shake. When she no longer could understand how to hold a sandwich, I would take the chicken out of the bread and fork or finger pieces of chicken to her. The milkshakes would sometimes work but was sometimes too thick, so she would try to scoop it out with her straw.

FTD robbing
My wife. Motor skills dropping
Ice cream on my shoes.

Smiling today but
Crying someday—aching for
love's endearing mishaps.

She would spill something and say, "Uh oh. You spilled."

I found it easier to just laugh and say, "Yes I did. I'm silly." I would wipe it off and continue our walk. She would get done with her milkshake, so I would simply carry it for her to let her focus. One thing at a time worked best.

We continued these walks and talks and occasional dances or twirls in the halls. She typically let me hold her close.

AFTD Social Media Post – 3/4/19

QUESTION: My wife's facility has a tiny chapel in it. Nobody was there tonight, so we went in, put on some Elvis, and danced. Are we going to hell?

Sarcasm did not always read well in print. Many readers tried to convince me not to worry about going to hell for dancing.

I never truly worried.

After the dance, I would return her to her routine of getting her into her pajamas and tucking her in. Then I would play soft music from my phone or her CD player in her room. She would drift off, and I would lean in with kisses, "I love you. Sweet dreams. Good night."

In her routine, she said nothing. I provided routines for her, not for me.

Sometimes, she changed that routine with a reply, "I love it when you are here."

Another case of the flu hit and interrupted our routines. Care facilities notoriously have to battle localized epidemics. With many residents in a fragile state, this can escalate into an emergency. Sadly, the residents get confused by it. They often do not understand explanations and protocols, and none more so than my wife in that condition.

I could still visit but had to mask and glove up and spend most of our time either in her room or out in the courtyard. Residents were typically locked down into the two halves (Tulip and Daffodil) to at least get one half of the population controlled against the virus. When someone became symptomatic, staff quarantined them to their room, which of course did not always last. They did not understand why they could not come out, even if told. Families often got called in to assist with that explanation, yet at the same time, they wanted to limit visitors to avoid a spread of the flu from outside.

Staff admittedly has a tough time enforcing a quarantine in facilities full of people with dementia.

Given Maureen's frail condition, I had them call me if they noticed anything out of the ordinary health-wise, no matter the time of day or night. I lived ten minutes away and worked thirty minutes away.

During that quarantine (nearly a year before the Coronavirus), Maureen did develop a fever. They called me at night with a 100.1 and a lot of oozing yellow discharge from the wound in her side. I had left her earlier that night feeling good. She had seemed alert and well. Apparently, the current virus around the facility attacked the gastro-intestinal system. Five of the thirty-six residents had it.

Hospice asked me if we should let nature take its course or get some antibiotics, since we had resigned to a "comfort, not cure" approach. I understood the question but thought something so easy to administer should happen without question. I would not quit on her. If nothing else, antibiotics would help with her comfort. I chose that. The nurse called it in, and I offered to go to the 24-hour pharmacist ten miles away to pick up the prescription so she could get started on it that night. With the pharmacy backed up with other prescriptions, I waited a couple of hours at a nearby all-night coffee house.

I returned. She woke up groggy but did open her eyes and see me. She said, "You're so beautiful. You're so nice." I found it both gentle and wonderfully odd how sometimes she could not form her thoughts and other times could. She took the medicine. I let her drift off now at nearly 1:00 in the morning. She smiled and even giggled a little—a happy sleep. How lovely.

Annie

She was lovely like lace
Yet comforting as tea,
But both are just things without soul,
And the depth of her soul was her greatest measure.

Her fever broke. Early March, even with that flu, she had shown herself more contented and even a little happier—seeming to be a bit more at peace.

Sometimes she would just sit with me on one of the couches and cuddle up against me, listening to her soft music. She just sat, relaxing and loving and content. Again, she seemed at peace.

Sometimes she would randomly kid around with an inside joke as she drank her Fanta, "They might be mad. I hope not. Too bad," and continue to drink and smile and giggle. She thought she got the better of something or someone. I had no idea who or what, but that did not matter. I liked to see her happy.

Despite our best attempts though, she continued to lose weight. It made me so sad. We could not force her to eat, and she did not want feeding tubes. Besides, in hospice, they do not offer feeding tubes as an option. Where we could get her a medicine or antibiotic, we did, but otherwise, we just made her comfortable. She still walked around, but everything really slowed down.

I would bring her fruit like mandarin oranges and watermelon because she would eat it, but it did nothing for putting weight on without the calorie count. I put a handful of chicken nuggets in my coat pocket and fed her as she paced. She usually ate them. That time of year, I could even try Girl Scout cookies. She could not resist Samoa's. Knowing the potential choking hazards with FTD, I fed those to her while she was seated and watched carefully. She never had a problem, except when we ran out. I brought several boxes.

To adjust to the weight loss, I picked up more and more pants and leggings. Her waist kept getting smaller. If I did not pay attention, the staff would cinch up her waistband in the back with a hair clip keeping it tight. I would go out that same day and get another few pairs of the next size down. I think that spring she got down to a size six. She eventually dropped to a size four.

I still tried to get her outside.

I found a memory garden fairly close by. A joint effort years earlier between the local government, the Alzheimer's Association, the Center of Design for an Aging Society, and others had this one constructed along with seven others around the country. They designed the garden circular to avoid getting lost and it was gated to avoid wandering off. Given their visitors were typically older or in wheelchairs, they planted flowers in raised beds. This made seeing and smelling the flowers easier for them. Maureen liked that garden in the spring as the first of the blooms started. We went often.

I had planned to take my Irish lass for a full picnic on St. Patrick's Day, but I could see, based on her mood that day, that these plans would not materialize. We adjusted again. I shifted those plans to taking her out for a milkshake and a brief stroll at the park. I never found the path uneven, but she struggled a bit and held my hand tightly—partly for tenderness and partly to steady herself. She smiled the whole time. I tried to keep her in the sun and not the shadows to keep her warm. It also made me sad, as I feared with her frailty, I would not get many more of these. I took a good picture with her, but my eyes welled up walking her back to the car and thought about how much I would miss those times.

She was now pacing less and sitting more. In fact, she lay down in bed a lot now—not wanting to get up. I would still get her out of bed each day just to keep her mobile. Her walking became labored. In the courtyard, she would trip on twigs on the ground and low curbs. She could no longer make one loop of the halls without sitting down to rest.

She also started to lose the mechanics of eating and drinking. Some nights, I begged her to drink her Ensure, but she would just hold the cup. Every time I tried to take her hand and bring it to her mouth, she would go rigid and would put the cup down. She left her stray white plastic Starbucks cups scattered around the halls—mostly untouched. The staff and I did our best all day long to get her to drink water so she would not dehydrate. I worried about FTD's aspirating pneumonia, given these mechanics breaking down.

Not even our go-to food options worked anymore: not the finger food meats and cheeses or even cookies. Some fruit still worked, but not enough to put the lost pounds back on. She had dropped below ninety pounds by the end of March, though they measured her at 92.4 at the beginning of the month.

She did not express any pain, but I still saw myself losing my baby.

At night, the closeness between us always remained as she lay in bed with me holding her hand. I would kiss it and gently brush her hair. I would tell her that I loved her and occasionally she would reciprocate, "I love love you baby." I kissed her, and her dry lips kissed me back a little. One night that month, her mind lucid for a few seconds, she looked directly at me and said, "I never never blame you."

Oh God. I blamed myself for not finding solutions to do more. I still do somedays.

I weep for you baby.

Scott's Journal – 3/19/19

This morning in a meeting, I received a call from a number that I did not know but thought it could be hospice—it was. Maureen was back to a low-grade fever and her wound very oozy, but they were able to get her out of bed and give her a little breakfast. I asked if it was imminent, and they said no, but it was not looking good. I finished up things in Ridgefield and made calls in prep to clear my schedule on my way to her and got there about 11:45. She sat staring at her lunch, not having taken a bite and nobody sitting with her to help.

Maureen delighted in seeing me and said, "Wow. What a surprise." I had just left her last night and took down her St. Patrick's decorations and put up spring tulips with a light Easter touch. Last night, she actually lay on her bed and watched me do it. She does not normally. She smiled and her eyes lit up, and I kept stopping and kissing her and telling her I loved her.

Today, she was so fragile that when I helped her from the lunch table to her room (where she said she wanted to go, as it was too noisy in the grand room), she tried to "air-sit" several times in that fifty steps to her room. I had to keep holding her up, as her weight was starting to go dead. I do not think she was collapsing as much as being tired, low energy, low strength, and just wanting to sit. I got her to her room and sat her down. Food is hard for her, so really none right now. She will drink water, but it has to be on her timing. If I force it, it will go in her lungs and cause her to cough, and then we could be talking aspiration pneumonia.

I sat with her a couple hours. A new hospice nurse, Jason, came and checked a few vitals. He let me know what I already knew and the hospice nurse had shared with me on the phone. "Maureen has no desire to eat or drink. This likely means she is approaching the end. I recommend soft foods like yogurt and pudding if she will have them. She does not seem to want to chew. I will tell staff." He left.

She did drink water with me a bit again on her own terms. She only had one swallow of the Ensure. I ran through her whole playlist as she lay there, sort of half-asleep, half just resting her eyes. She seemed stable, so I left and came back about 5:15 so I could do some paperwork and get caught up without that hanging over me.

She was in the same position, lying there. I came in and she recognized my voice with her eyes closed. Sometimes she opened them and sometimes not. She said things in and out of a sleep that had nothing to do with reality and then drifted off again. Sometimes she opened her eyes and saw me. I told her I loved her. Most times she was quiet but smiled. Other times she mustered, "Yeah."

She hummed to music. It was lighter, more ethereal, like she was floating. She said she was sick in the stomach and did not want anything, but did not express pain either. They checked on her hourly. Sometimes we just let her sleep in her clothes. They would change her to her pajamas if she woke up later but did not want to agitate her.

Holding her hand at her bedside, I part wept and part marveled. She heard my words. Sometimes she responded with a few unrecognizable words and sometimes silence. It did not matter. She was gentle and good and kind and loving and simply the embodiment of those things.

> I was just floating in a way too. I felt as though I had no control of my movements and just wafting back and forth in this breeze of life, this wind of uncertainty.
>
> My heart aches for times squandered.

AFTD Social Media Post – 3/30/19

Dance more in the sunshine. Laugh more in the moment. Kiss more in the open. Some days, FTD can be everything—most days, make it nothing.

Rest. My precious rest

Simply—void of the weary

Race I would run for you.

Rest from making sense

No need my wife.

Let deeply buried dreams loose

Tonight, so you might soar.

Rest, rest joyously.

The days of April passed swiftly with this excruciating routine of Maureen near death, then rallying, then dying again. The days truly blended into weeks. Everything seemed to fly by yet remain utterly on hold. I initiated nothing, it seemed. I waited and reacted. I had never felt so out of control of events around my life. I wondered how she felt that month, lying there so ill and so weak.

My baby's physical condition had not changed significantly—seemingly stabilizing on the brink. She had multiple temperature spikes. At one point, they had to put her in isolation (she had not gotten out of bed much anyway) because she had diarrhea and a fever. The staff still had to protect the other residents from contagious viruses. They stuck the PPE box outside her door for the staff's protection. The illness passed, apparently not what they had feared. They removed the box three days later.

She developed a red spot next to her wound that we watched—worried it would become a second hole to bandage.

I had read that fluctuating temperatures could signal "the end"—your body stops regulating itself. I feared so much for her when that end time would come. Would she feel ready? Would I know and sit there with her or would it happen in the still of night? Would she awake and realize it and wonder where I went or have me there and wonder why I could not fix it? I agonized over it but always reminded myself that she agonized more.

I thought about the issue of why we hold on to our loved ones with terminal conditions. If we loved them, we would let them go—right? Perhaps we know they want life, not death, and we want for them what they want for themselves. They may not want to leave yet. They may just want a life free of pain, a life back to what they had before. However, I know it cannot go back. So why not let go? The paradox: feeling selfish for helping her.

In some way, I had let her go by bringing in hospice four months earlier and entering this comfort mode, rather than curative. I asked myself if she kept choosing to hang on.

I hope she did not think about me later and wonder why I did not help her pass more quickly or question any of the treatment I had provided for her. I did my best. We had not prepared for dementia.

She had no real family history of it. Why would we think it would happen to us?

I think most caregivers agonize over these questions. You can do some things to pragmatically prepare for what you know is coming, which may free you up to emotionally take in the moment without the burden of asking, "What should I have done?" or "What should I do now?" Some tips for well ahead of this moment:

1. Have healthcare directives in place.

2. Put a trust, will, and durable power of attorney in place.

3. Know their wishes for after they die.

4. Know the funeral home that you want to use to receive their body (not necessarily where the service itself will take place).

5. Call people you think would want to see your loved one a last time and respect their wishes if they do not.

6. Create a contact list of key people in your loved one's friend and family tree and rely on those people to spread the word.

7. Write down your thoughts for all the good they brought to this world. You may be overcome with grief later and cannot get to that place.

8. Share this information with someone else so they can help ease your burdens after. Don't sit alone.

9. Tell yourself there is no need to rush afterward. If you need more time, take it.

No matter the preparation, emotionally it will not matter. When you love someone so deeply and they pass, you will react the same as if you had not prepared at all.

I did not want to artificially extend her life of pain. I just wanted to take care of this life of hers. I simply wanted to care for her life here in the most loving way I could. Time and inevitability would determine the moment that she went, and I would mourn and grieve for quite some time. As I should and knew I would.

AFTD Social Media Post – 4/14/19

Fair or not, smiles or sobs, cream or crap, we'll keep being there—not just because it's the right thing to do, but because we're the ones that love them most. Good luck this week.

She certainly hunched over more, tired more, rested more, and paced so very little. She took to standing and rocking back and forth rather than making the hallway trips that she used to. Perhaps she got so disoriented that she thought she still walked the halls. She started to complain of pain. As such I asked them to monitor that more closely. They had her up to Hydromorphone on eight-hour doses but could also provide a lighter dose on the hour if the pain intensified.

She still took the Mirtazapine for the anti-depressant mood stabilizer and the Melatonin at night to help her sleep through the night.

While I resisted drugs myself, if it gave her comfort and kept her on a routine, then I welcomed it. I had always researched the side effects of medications to make the most informed choices for my wife. Mirtazapine could cause constipation, so they had a stool softener on hand, but they rarely used it.

Mentally, she continued to deteriorate. I did not know where she would find bottom. Would she hit that before the cancer took her? She had recognized people less, communicated less, and understood less. She had a few mood swings, but not many. She just seemed completely spent most of the time. I still brought her mother to see her weekly, but often Maureen hardly even acknowledged her presence, which must have taken its toll on her mother emotionally.

Added to that, Maureen's red spot a few inches from her first wound had opened up, so she had a second wound site. Oddly, she did not seem to take notice. Maybe because they sat so close together, and they already regularly bandaged one, another simply went beyond her notice. We all became far more concerned than her and continued efforts to make her comfortable.

Again, Maureen seemed spent and so very tired. She had fewer lucid moments and was in a fog so often. She could not lie on the bed and scoot herself up to her pillows to sit or even lean much anymore. I had taken to lifting her and scooting her back. She used to balk, but rarely did that anymore. I think she had resigned to her fate. It made me so sad.

I would sit with Maureen for long periods, sometimes in silence, just letting her rest and holding her hand. She grasped my hand tightly. I moved it periodically on purpose just so she would react and hold it tighter. Her reaction told me that she remained awake despite the closed eyes and still knew I sat with her, holding her.

But then overnight, mid-month, I arrived at the facility, and she had rallied. I found her walking in the grand room—this amazing and strong woman. She held on as though she had more to say or do.

I called that our miracle morning. I came in and saw her slowly walking around and exclaimed, "Honey. Sweetie. Maureen." She looked up and had such a glorious smile and look of recognition on her face. She stretched out her arms for a hug. She stood still, so I came to her. It made me well up. I hugged her long and tight. I loved this moment that I had not seen for weeks. We walked a little and sat and listened to some music that she hummed to a lot. She loved her music. Later that day after my departure and return, that energy waned slightly. No matter the staff levels, they could never provide one-on-one engagement for more than a few minutes.

She heard me and grinned and hobbled to get up. I supported her. They had left her jacket on. Her cheeks were flushed, and that heat always impacted her thinking. We struggled to get her jacket off and carried her to her bed. I propped up her pillows so she could sit back and not hunch over so deeply. We had established a routine: the jacket on in the morning and off in the afternoon. I tried to get the staff to understand that (sigh). I gave her a drink of water but had to hold it for her to get a few sips. Per the hospice nurse, I did not force it, but let her sip from only a slight tilt.

Prior to the joy of that day, I cared for my soul with outdoor walks at the Foster Floodplain, writing poetry and drinking tea. Typically, midday Saturdays, I would go to this little place called Cup of Tea and just order a small pot and a snack and sit and read to restore a sense of me. One such Saturday, I had rolled the paperback into my back pocket, and a lady who worked there asked what I had done with my book, so I presented it. I laughed and asked if I had developed a reputation. She said she had noticed that I came there to quietly read and recharge and take some time for me—all as a positive.

Yes, I found it important to take care of myself as I took care of Maureen SO that I could take care of Maureen. Everyone told me that, and I relented to its truth. I still felt guilty sometimes and would cut it short to race back to her.

This habit helped give me strength as I walked the path with the love of my life. I had mentally and emotionally "buried" Maureen several times in the last few months every time a doctor or nurse would say, "This is the end." I decided I could no longer do that—keep burying Maureen. I prepared again, rallied myself again, to simply find the joy in whatever small moments we had left and keep looking to the positive.

I knew that her passing would devastate me. However, I was tired of getting devastated every couple of days. I cried most days, but thought I simply had to solider on. I reminded myself, again, that I had the opportunity to still treasure our moments together. Again, my march never compared to hers. She battled with herself daily in what must have felt like a tug of war with madness.

I loved her every day and every moment. By allowing myself the space sometimes to let her mind rest and renew my connection with her after a few hours away, I could savor this time. I still saw her every day, two to three times a day—not out of obligation, rather love. I knew time with her would make good memories that I would carry with me long after she passed.

Though she remained tired, she did get better. I never imagined somebody could rally as much as her. I would look at her and smile and lean in for a kiss, and she would lift her hand and cup my cheek, pulling me in and holding it there for a while. She stared at me and stalled on the next step—just sort of frozen in that moment. What a glorious moment for time to stand still. I kept seeing the magnificence in the ordinary.

At night, when I left her lying in her bed with her eyes closed and said that I would come back tomorrow, she would grin, still with her eyes closed. It provided me some sort of affirmation that she was content. Again, "magnificence in the ordinary."

To honor this most recent rally, I continued to train up the newly arriving staff to help me. One of Maureen's favorite med-aids had left, as did a couple of her preferred caregivers. We managed. I had renewed vigor and a second wind, but oh how they tried my patience.

I would find her in her room bundled up and hot. I would strip off the blankets and open her window and door to get a cross breeze going. I had warned them that the first indicator when she got too warm included flushed cheeks. "Watch for that," I reminded (sigh).

On a Thursday morning before I brought her mother, I swung in to check on her state of mind. They had her sitting with a bib eating breakfast at a table with three men. She did not know them nor had she ever sat with them before. Nobody spoke (not even the normally chatty men), and nobody looked comfortable (again, not even the men). She did not need a bib. She needed feeding assistance. You use a bib when one feeds themselves but has lost some of that dexterity. In her state, she would never grab that spoon.

I removed the bib and took her for a walk to the other side of the day room, and she grinned and got very chatty again. The staff's lack of attention frustrated me. On her schedule that they had, every Thursday, they had to get her ready by 9:30 for her mother. Ready meant done and waiting for us and not sitting with a bunch of men making her uncomfortable. She had trust issues with strangers. I kept thinking, "Read the damn write up I gave you."

I took a breath but remained passionate about this rally, and I did not want to see her slide backwards.

Her visit with her mom that day went as well as it could. Maureen stayed pretty alert and seemed to recognize her mom, sort of. Her mother said, "Hello sweetheart. It's your momma."

Maureen would only respond, "Uh huh." As such, her mother had to assume Maureen knew what she meant.

In the car home, she started to analyze a couple things Maureen did and tried identifying causes. I understood the impulse but explained again to her as I had many times before, "I understand you want to explain it or identify a cause other than FTD. I know that you want someone to just do "this or that," and we can permanently fix it for always. Believe me, I do too. Please understand that it is nothing different that you did today, or I did. The behavior is random, and her responses to the same situations can differ drastically hour to hour or day-to-day. There is no logic to it. We just have to ride it out each time. The more you try to fix it, the more frustrated you will be the next time when she doesn't respond the same way."

She commented that Maureen had flinched a little, so she had asked Maureen if she made her nervous, and she replied, "Yeah." She just laughed and said that Maureen told her that as a kid too. "I guess I still do. I don't know why." I did not take that huge invitation but instead chose to remain silent. I knew her mother was hurting, and I had no need to bring up decades of issues. Maybe some other time in the distant future, or not at all.

I focused on Maureen's rally and tried to stoke it.

I had brought her fresh flowers each week since she moved to the facility. I trimmed them in front of her and placed them in a favorite small purple vase of hers. More alert with this rally, she watched me do it and commented the whole time. I handed her one of the flowers and asked her, "Smell this one honey."

"Well it smells beautiful," she said, then dismissively tossed it on the floor, "But it's gone."

I said nothing but picked up the flower and included it in the bouquet. After a pause looking out the window, she turned toward the bouquet and said with a smile, "Beautiful."

FTD does a to-and-fro most days.

In the timing of these improved moments for us, the administrator of the AFTD social site, Lauren, reached out to me to see if I would speak as a panelist for social media storytelling—a breakout session at their annual conference held in Los Angeles that year. I initially said "no" to stay with Maureen, but as I looked at the itinerary, I saw that they structured it as only a one-day conference, so I could fly in Thursday night, do the conference, and fly home Friday night and still see Maureen both days.

As such, I told her yes, but I reserved my prerogative to reassess closer to the time. With six panelists, if I had to cancel the trip last minute due to Maureen's health, they would manage easily. Public speaking gave me neither concern nor pride (I had done that plenty in my career); however, the connection with the FTD community and sharing Maureen's story did excite me. I could see myself championing this cause and telling her story long after my beloved passed.

They held the conference in May, a couple of weeks after a much more special event: Maureen's sixty-ninth birthday.

AFTD Social Media Post – 4/28/19

BIRTHDAY BALANCE

My beautiful bride persevered to see her sixty-ninth birthday yesterday. This provided me such joy, knowing all she has gone through this last three years. She smiled much of the day, though also tired easily.

I repeated prior themes: preparation, keeping it small, and flexibility. Outings also require calm music, familiar surroundings, and low activity. Her weakened state makes for short walks with a lot of sitting to listen and look.

I purchased a few decorations, lunch, and dessert the day before and placed it all before picking her up. I set an elongated schedule, allowing far more time than needed.

We got her Starbucks at a drive through, drove to our park with windows rolled down drinking and listening to her music, went to our old house with simple decorations, her favorite barbeque pulled pork and potato salad followed by her favorite cake and ice cream—all small portions.

I read her cards from friends and family as she cannot read anymore and had her pull new clothes out of a birthday bag (unwrapping is hard for her).

She ate well, and we sway-danced to Elvis, The Beatles, Peter, Paul, and Mary, and others. She then got sleepy, so I lay her down on our old bed for a short nap while I picked up things before returning her to her facility. We spent four hours, with minor missteps along the way, but she had a good time.

Things I learned:

- Her vision is so poor and her gait so restricted that our stairs are now a problem for her to see and understand to lift her foot.

- I need to read the package better for the banner to avoid, "Happy 1st Birthday" (I carefully cut the middle out).

- I need to worry less about her spilling her drink and more about ME spilling her drink. "Uh oh—you made a mess," she said. I could only chuckle.

- Our fewer outings cause things to be a bigger deal for her. "Oh crap—that's a mess," she said. "What dear—the cars?" I asked. "Yeah, that's a lot of cars." There were three.

- I need to listen to what everyone says about taking care of myself—I was dragging.

This last one is hard for me, because to do that, I take a break from FTD—she never gets to take a break from FTD. The guilt can weigh heavily, but finding that peace is essential.

When I was single, I used to go to the Portland Japanese Gardens for that peace—that recentering. While we went a few times during our marriage, I did not need to go, as she created my peace. While there will always be love and tenderness, FTD does not allow her the words and the touch and the intention to create that peace anymore.

As such, I went back to the gardens today. I still marvel at the forms of water and the symbolism. The babbling brook has calms and rushes representative of our day-to-day lives. The cascade or waterfalls represent the extremes in our lives that we must weather. The still pond is our calm, our restoration, our peace we seek for ourselves. "He leads me beside still waters…"

I went to Maureen before the gardens. I had laid out her new birthday clothes for the caregivers to put on her—reminiscent of her bohemian/hippy days—a flowered tunic and frayed capris. She smiled.

Now after my return, we walked and held hands. I reminded her of her birthday events yesterday and asked if she had a nice birthday. She said, "Yeah." I was back to my joy but now had balance.

Her behavioral crashes or outbursts had stopped by that spring—her most intense were from fall 2017 to fall 2018. I never knew whether to credit the mood stabilizing Mirtazapine or simply something she had progressed out of. On occasion, she still had a minor and brief outburst associated with one of her triggers—like getting too hot.

One afternoon a few days after her birthday, I found her sitting alone in her room. I asked her to stand up and take a walk with me out in the courtyard, as it was a beautiful day. With her labored walking, I helped her outside.

We eventually sat down in the gazebo, and she truly enjoyed our time together. The sun had passed over the chair she sat in, so it was very warm. While we were only out for a short time, she started to get too warm. I tried to bring her in, but she really did not want to get up—maybe partially due to her physical limitations and partially because the sun felt good on her face. Her cheeks had gotten flushed though, and I did not want to risk her getting overheated, as she easily did.

Once inside and back on a familiar couch, she turned on me and called me a "bastard" and "liar". The heat had gotten to her. I had failed to act in time. I told her "Honey. I am sorry. I was just trying to help you." She got quiet for a while and looked down as though she had to think on that prospect. She did not insist she had "to go" as she had before. She did not continue to rage at me. Truthfully, she did not even obsess over some small object around her. She just got quiet, like she was deep in thought.

I waited a bit and then held her hand. She let me and placed her other hand on mine. She continued to look down, but I knew she had quickly snapped out of the worst of it. As I said before, she tossed those "soft needles" at me sometimes. No harm done. She could not control what the FTD did to her, like watching herself in a movie. FTD causes an emotional pain in that they often know what they did—they would see themselves do it, but could only watch, like a bystander in their own life.

I could see it made her sad. I said I loved her, and she grinned. She knew she had not hurt me.

Still hesitant to leave her for even a day for the AFTD conference in Los Angeles, I made the flight. She seemed stable. I caught a 2 p.m. flight that Thursday and went back on an 8:00 p.m. flight on Friday. I made her my last stop before leaving and my first stop when I returned.

I wanted to share her story, but I also wanted to learn what more I could do for Maureen. I looked in on her after 11:00 that night, driving from the airport to her side. I just expected to watch her sleep for a bit. I kissed her on the forehead and said softly, "I love you." With eyes still closed, she grinned and said, "Mm-hmm." I found that enough. Whatever she could give me I found enough.

Scott's Journal – 5/5/19

I am sitting here late in the evening alone on our old deck and typing about my wife, wishing for her to actually be sitting here next to me instead. The frogs croak in the background. Of course I was there multiple times today—three times: morning, midday, and evening to tuck her in. I take extra time during the weekend.

Tonight, I got there about 7:15, and they had got her pajamas on, but she was still awake. They ran out of the Melatonin. How do you do that? Do an inventory and order it.

Anyway, I did my, "Ta-da! It's you husband!" She glanced up and grinned.

I cuddled up next to her on the tiny bed and gave her kisses and held her gently. She started to make a few short, noun-less comments that had no meaning or clarity that I could understand, as is typical now. It is that, or silence. I grabbed onto a word or two and repeated it back to her as though I understood, which seemed to satisfy her. She lay there quietly then. There is a part of her that wants to communicate, though unable to, and there is another part of her that just wants to curl up into a ball and disappear.

I gave her some Fanta as she likes. I also gave her some water and some of her Ensure. It was too cold in the room, so I turned the AC to just the fan mode to keep the airflow.

We listened to many songs on her playlist—her softly humming to most of them. Part of the time I sat next to her bed and held her hand, and other parts I cuddled up, spooning behind her a little, just so she could feel my presence. Also, I suppose so I could feel hers.

She does not like to walk a lot anymore and really struggles, but the staff did get her out of bed today and to a table for lunch. It was a nice day out, but she seemed pretty tired, so I did not push it. I will try again for a brief walk outside with her tomorrow. I need to watch closely and switch her to a wheelchair if she continues to struggle. A conversation with hospice is needed for her safety.

There is so little muscle left, just skin and bones—and hardly a cliché in her case. I rub my hand down her hip when she lies on her side, and I am ever so gentle because I feel the hip bone and the thigh bone as opposed to the supple hips and thighs she had before. My eyes well up again—been doing that a lot this weekend.

Last night, I sat next to her as she lay in bed and told her I loved her (I tell her that many times a day), and while in the last four to six weeks she has rarely responded in kind like she used to, she surprised me. She quietly said, "I love you my life." I knew what she meant, and the tears rolled down my cheeks. I said back to her, constraining the lump in my throat, "I love you my life too." After a moment, she looked right at me with her own eyes, not the vacant ones, and said, "We had life fun."

Oh God! I looked down and squeezed my eyes shut as though my lids were sponges to sop up the tears (did not work) and choked out, "Yes, we had fun baby—lots of fun."

I rattled off places we had travelled to and concerts we had seen. When I got to Disneyland, she said, "Yeah, I liked that." That was the last trip we took. We strolled as though we were the only ones in that magical park.

I reminded her of It's a Small World and the Tiki Room and then found those theme songs on my phone. She hummed along as always. I miss those trips with her. That was just a year ago, and she could walk, look around, take things in, and talk. It was not always the words that she wanted, but enough. That was before the next mental descent and before the cancer.

Scott's Journal – 5/6/19

Today I brought small mandarin oranges and offered one to Maureen. She was delighted. We sat down. I was on her bed and she in her chair (role reversal from the norm). I peeled it and, slice by slice, fed it to her. She never wavered and enjoyed them fully. I never had to convince her to open her mouth or remind her we were eating. I put the others in her fridge.

She was in a walking mood today, which was nice, so we walked slowly from one room to another, would sit a spell, and then continue on again. She would sit on a couch, and I would drop to the floor so she could see me directly, since she hangs her head almost always now. I hold her hand, and we just sit there looking at each other.

Before I left to return to work, I asked to kiss her, and she did not respond, so I settled for the forehead. After I did that, she asked, "Do you do that everywhere?" I was not sure what she meant, but took it at face value and replied, "No. I only kiss you. You're the only one I kiss." That must have nailed it because she looked up and smiled and puckered. I obliged and received a "Yeah."

I returned in the evening after a phone call from the med-aid that Maureen had fallen in her room. There was a water glass on the floor. They were not sure if she slipped or fell or perhaps went to sit and misjudged. They completely checked her out and saw no bruises or anything. Maureen did not complain of pain nor act as though she had any pain. She sat herself back on the bed. She may have tried to "air-sit". We will never know what happened.

While her language skills are rapidly declining, so is her thought process. She cannot figure most things out. She cannot initiate nearly anything. She struggles to reason anything. She wanders and must be led. The world is too big of a place for her, and she cannot manage alone most activities that we take for granted.

I see others in her care facility, and while there are a few somewhat bad off, most just go on day-to-day. Little seems wrong with them, except their memory going and getting easily confused. They still function. I see and live the difference between Alzheimer's and FTD with Maureen.

Maureen bites or kisses a straw as much as she sucks on it. She holds things in her hand with no idea what to do with it next. She compulsively grabs folds of fabric of her clothing or a neighboring blanket. She wanders without purpose, or any purpose we understand. She may in fact be searching, but for what we do not know.

I offered her a Fanta today, and she said a loud "YES" immediately after I finished the last syllable, and then followed it up with, "That was a good yes."

I laughed—yes it was. I said, "You like those Fantas, huh?"

She replied, "Yeah. They're cheap." I smiled—not the adjective I expected. "They're...just...purple," she continued. The paraphasia of her FTD replaced her "perfect". I never, ever correct. I would rather have the word salad than no words at all.

I brought along with the oranges, some smaller pants—trying size fours now as the sixes almost fall off her. She seemed ok from what we thought was a fall. I told the med-aid to connect with hospice about a wheel-chair, as it seemed it was time, and I did not want her hurting herself. The challenge would be whether she would think to stay sat in it or not. I still thought it best to have on hand.

We talked and walked a bit and listened to her music. I checked her for bruises or any trauma and saw nothing. I slow danced with her a bit in the halls and entry to the chapel.

At one point, near her room, she said, "You're so nice. You're so great." That felt good.

Later I rubbed her exposed calf below the capri pants, and she said that felt "really nice". I take these wins, as we might go several days without another.

> I lay her down tonight and let her fall asleep. I cuddled a little with her for just a song. She smiled as I parted the same as always, "I love you baby. Good night. Sweet dreams. I love you always."

Caregiving can take a lot of time, but it is so worthwhile for her joy and comfort. However, other responsibilities tend to pile up. Our beautiful house had sat on the market for nine months without an offer, but the days started to get longer and sunnier. I knew our house showed best in the spring, so I remained optimistic. We got it featured in a home magazine and increased the open houses.

Sadly, we had depleted all our savings and started going into debt. I tightened everywhere I could, but FTD with this level of care can drain your finances. I had no resentment, nor regrets. I would never move her or reduce her care. If things got really bad, I could take out an equity loan.

With those sunnier May days, Maureen's spirits seemed to buoy.

I would take her out into the courtyard for a walk. With no wind initially, I asked her if she enjoyed it. She nodded, as she used few words these days. Then a gentle breeze came in, and she immediately acted cold, even with her jacket still on. She said nothing but sounds. I would convince her to make one more trip around the courtyard before going back in. She then, with the wind still gently blowing, smiled again, and felt fine. Her mind must just race all the time. Do not let anyone ever tell you that FTD just stops a person's mind. No, she constantly tried to figure things out.

That spring I brought more fruit: grapes, mandarin oranges, and watermelon. While I knew these did not get her the calories she needed, I also knew she would eat them. The most calorie-dense foods in the world did not matter if she only took a bite. Typically, she ate almost all the fruit that I brought. I found myself even bringing a little extra fruit for one of the other residents that had worked as a nurse much earlier in her life. Now in her nineties, she would stop me most visits to ask about Maureen. She also commented how the facility served mostly processed food. They even served fruit cocktail instead of pieces of fruit. She missed whole fruit. She spent her days bound to a wheelchair and had Alzheimer's but remained quite alert. I would slip her the occasional orange or clump of grapes.

During daytime naps or evenings when Maureen stayed particularly quiet, I just sat in her chair next to her bed for a bit and watched her breathe. I would look around her room. The furniture and art that I had placed there rekindled memories of our time together. Maureen had selected the two chairs in her room some thirteen years earlier for the new house. We had used them along our bedroom picture window to look out over the trees and East Portland with coffee or tea. I remembered her feeling particularly proud of that find.

For the corner I had chosen our antique tea cart that she had discovered under three vintage suitcases in a consignment shop: Victorian and in great shape—another great find. It just needed a little cleaning. I never would have noticed it, but she caught the walnut color out of the corner of her eye. We now used it to support her mini fridge of drinks and snacks as well as a vase of fresh flowers I would replenish each week.

Her nightstand came from a more modern, Mission collection that we had bought as an unfinished pair. She had stained it with a nutmeg color two years before we built our new home. We finished it together, and that made her smile. Little did I realize she had envisioned our home and its colors long before we even bought the site. I laughed thinking about the thirty-six doors, forty-two windows, and what seemed like miles of wood trim that we prepped, stained, and varnished for our beautiful home. We enjoyed that time together—work or play.

It now held her snack basket that I kept stocked, a small CD player for care staff to use with her, and three photo albums with everything labelled for her. The labeling, while well intentioned, may have not mattered much. She never initiated looking at the albums. I would use them to talk about our adventures together. She could only read a few words anymore, but perhaps some words as we turned the pages together still made sense.

Throughout May, she walked less and less, and hospice had prepared me that she may just stop one day. They put a Geri chair and wheelchair on standby to have on hand when it seemed unsafe for her to walk.

Some days though, she would still surprise and delight me.

I would come in and she would behave more alertly than normal. The staff would tell me, "Maureen walked a lot on her own today. It was a good day." For her to take the initiative to walk represented a small victory to celebrate. I often found her in the grand room sitting with a caregiver. The caregiver would see me and signal to Maureen that I had arrived. She would look up kind of to the side with her head still hung and see me, smile, and say, "Oh my gosh. I cannot believe him. So surprised." I always came in for a hug and kiss.

Her limited walking that month paled in comparison to the frantic pacing from before. Her gait kept very slow and measured, but it was still a positive for sure. She used my hand to steady herself, since we still held hands frequently. We had that as our thing. Those public displays of affection during our marriage would make the grandchildren go, "Ewww", thus encouraging us to do it all the more.

Mid-month toward the end of an afternoon visit, she was sitting on the edge of the bed facing the window but looking down. I came up next to her and sort of lay on the bed on my stomach and came up to her right side and looked at her, though she had not looked up or at me. I told her, "I love you." She smiled slightly and nodded. A reciprocal "I love you" had not occurred for a few weeks, as so many words had disappeared. I chose to prompt her and asked, "Do you love me?"

She turned and looked at me with her original eyes—not the ones FTD had left her with, but restored for a fleeting moment to a knowledgeable, caring, and aware person. She stared right into my soul and said, "I have loved you a long time, a very long time." That just stopped me cold. I said, "Thank you, baby." I hugged her waist and she leaned down and kissed the top of my head. She then looked away and hummed and asked me, "Are you you married?"

I said, "Yes. I'm married to you baby." I said it softly, trying to bring her back.

She did not react. She absently held my hand and then looked down and studied it and turned it over back and forth and looked up to my elbow. "That's Scott," she said.

"Yes, it IS me baby."

"Good," she said and went back to humming and continued holding my hand.

You take the good and the bad and the odd all together. I do not think she forgot me as much as tried to sort out her thoughts. It saddened me, nonetheless. I could not even remember the last time she used my name.

Sometimes though, in my car, I would sit alone in the driveway or at the back of a parking lot and just scream at the injustice. I made sure though, to always detach anything negative from Maureen and to never categorize her as this "FTD person". Alone, I imagined myself with Maureen, healthy and sitting next to me, staring at how

FTD had left her. Would she cry with me? Would she need a hug from me? Would she simply accept it as some sort of fate?

Try as I might, I could not empathize with her hell. I had not lived in her shoes. I could not lead her to the fix. It left me both sad and frustrated. However, those frustrations at the injustices meant I still passionately clung to her. I still loved her deeply. I felt helplessness and sorrow every day.

I forced myself daily to find something to smile about. While feeding Maureen I would tell her "good job" after a bite, and she would respond wryly, "Yes it was." I could smile at that. I knew that in the near future, she might stop talking, and I would have to look back on that moment to find my smile.

You have to look hell in the eye and find something to celebrate when you really just want to scream.

That Mother's Day weekend, her son came up with his wife the day before. Maureen generally stayed in an ok mood and receptive to their visit, though I think her understanding of the who and why of visitors had mostly left her. I felt for her son and wife and the loss they likely felt. Maureen's daughter and family came the next day as part of an errand in Portland.

That morning, the facility had a brunch, and she did fair but was really agitated. The noise and break from routine and the people and the bustle became just too much for her. She preferred the norm. In fact, earlier that week, she had made the comment, "You're so nice. You're so calm." While I would not know what to do with that compliment from others, from her, it made total sense: she equated calm to happiness. When she felt calm, she could articulate more and share those feelings and find her words.

Her mother wanted to keep making her weekly trips but understandably got disappointed in how little Maureen acknowledged her. Her mother tried to connect, but only as much as she knew how. She would not take pointers from me. She would only stay in her own comfort zone. At eighty-nine, I could not expect change, and I understood that.

She also refused to do any personal soul searching as to why she did not have that strong connection with Maureen. I did not think that I should try to explain it to her. She could not fix it anyway. She teared up a bit at the end of most visits, or even during. She wanted a closer relationship with Maureen—to come into the room and receive immediate recognition and warmth. Now, however, she no longer had the time to try and fix decades of missed cues. That window had shut.

Maureen's apathy became more frequent, which often develops as a part of FTD. Her mother said, "She just does not remember me, or she does not care."

I sat with her mother again and shared calmly, "FTD is not a memory disease. She does remember. She just cannot always access the memories or sort her thoughts. Yes, it is very likely that often she does not care that you are here." This obviously bothered her. I further explained what we had discussed many times previously, "Apathy is a part of FTD. The part of her brain that does sympathy and empathy is atrophied. She will come off as apathetic or even callous sometimes. You have to understand that all of this is the FTD, not her. If she could reason it, she would tell you she loved you."

"Well I just think she doesn't remember me," she retorted, getting out of the car at her apartment.

Later in FTD, people can develop some memory challenges, and Maureen certainly had progressed in this disease. But these vacant expressions from Maureen had gone on for a while. I knew her mother was hurting and trying to reason through it. I guess I just did not know what to say.

The visits had not always ended distant and sorrowful for her and her mother. Late May they had a beautiful moment. I would typically see Maureen in the morning before I picked up her mother to make sure staff had Maureen ready and that she generally seemed receptive—prepping if you will. I walked with Maureen a bit and took her to the side room couch. She seemed ok. I left her there to go get her mother. When we returned, we went to that same spot, and not only had Maureen stayed there, she had put up her feet on the couch, laid back, and relaxed as though she didn't have a care in the world.

I let her mother lead to the couch and engage her.

"Hello sweetheart. It's your mother."

"Why yes. Yes, it is," Maureen replied.

They exchanged hugs and her mother followed with, "How are you feeling today?"

Maureen launched into a word salad narrative that absolutely tickled her as she told the story. She sat close to her mother like a good girlfriend and just shared this adventure that we could make neither heads nor tails of. She got the giggles, which in turn gave her mother the giggles. After this much time, her mother seemed to finally understand not to ask Maureen what she meant, but to simply receive it. I had brought a latte for her mother and a chai tea latte for Maureen, and they just sat and giggled and had a grand time—a good trip for her mother to have.

Afterward, at the request of the caregiving staff, I had the in-house hair stylist cut Maureen's hair by three to four inches to get rid of the split ends, so her beautiful long blond hair would grow healthier and get less tangled.

Maureen hung in there like a trooper. I prepared for her to fight it or get fidgety, but she just sat still—no problems. She hung her head the whole time, so the stylist changed her approach for a drooping head. It looked great, and the caregivers said they had a much easier time now brushing her hair. I agreed as we took turns brushing—something I had started back when we first dated. She had such beautiful hair.

She started struggling more physically by late in the month. The walking became such a challenge. I would walk her out facing her (me walking backwards) with both of my hands on both of hers and her hunched over. She collapsed. I caught her before she went to the floor—a slow descent though, almost like she started searching for a chair. She had lightly fallen three times in three weeks—they thought. Three times they had gone in her room and found her sitting on the floor—no scratches, no bruises, no pain. They did not know for sure but suspected.

We got a chair to her, and they immediately started asking her if she needed her wheelchair. I thought, "Relax people. Let her breathe. Let her pause and collect." I sat on the floor so I could make eye contact with her on the chair looking down. I stayed there for a long while offering reassuring words. I asked her, "Honey. Would you like me to get you a chai tea?"

"I will come," she replied. I had not intended that, but I thought, "We'll try." I took both of her hands again and helped her up. She resumed walking. We got to the car (parked right at the entry) and struggled a little to get her in. She would not get in as normal, so I turned her toward me and sat her down, then spun her legs in, and then did her seatbelt as I always did.

I of course played her music, got our teas, and found a little spot at a park. I rolled down the windows, and we stayed in the car. She enjoyed her tea, though she was a bit confused: she started feeling for the small hole in the lid with her tongue as she had always done, but almost like someone blind. She had not turned the cup right, but FTD kept her from reasoning to turn the cup. As such, she drank with her hand at an odd, backwards-like angle. I knew better then to straighten it for her as she would feel I took it away. We still had a wonderful time sitting in the quiet, drinking together, and enjoying soft tunes.

I brought her back, and her walking remained labored. She needed to sit down twice before making it back to her room. Fearful for her safety, I decided we could no longer wait on the mobile chairs. I flagged down the med-aid and asked her to get hospice to bring the Geri chair and said I would bring an already purchased wheelchair with me later that day. We had bought one previously for her mother when she had knee pain. Her mother would not use it. "Fine," I thought. Maureen would now use it instead.

That same month, we had arranged to replace her standard bed with a mechanical, adjustable bed. It made it easier for us to get her comfortable. With so much loss of muscle, the better mattress and alternate positions better cradled her poor bones. This bed also made it easier for her to eat and drink in bed as she became prone to do more since the walking had become more difficult. The inclined position also helped her to swallow safely.

While she had gotten much quieter these days, sometimes words in her mind would just align. I think when they did, she just needed to say them to get them out. Just off the cuff one morning I sat there, and she said, "I'm perfect. I'm perfect."

I laughed and said, "Yes you are perfect."

She said, "Yeah."

I do not know where that came from. We had just listened to "I Got You Babe" by Sonny and Cher. She often repeated words, but they did not say "perfect" in the song. I delighted in watching how emphatically she said it.

Later that same day she looked down at herself while lying on the bed and exclaimed, "I have no zippers. How embarrassing."

She motioned at her clothing. I could scarcely remember a time in many months that she had used a noun without me saying it first.

I said, "You know, I have no zippers either."

She replied, "Oh, ok," and all seemed fine. I had never thought of the lack of zippers as embarrassing. An FTD mind races.

A caregiver came in to talk to me about Maureen's activities of the day. They had this habit of talking about Maureen in front of her rather than to her. A quick statement or two was fine, but when they went on and on, I tried (unsuccessfully) to redirect them toward Maureen. Too much talking, too busy and not toward her would make her agitated.

I would balance their debriefs between listening and trying to make eye contact with Maureen or at least rubbing her hand. I wanted her to stay engaged. This happened while Maureen was lying there in the bed after the zipper embarrassment. The caregiver finally left, and I made the comment to Maureen, "Boy she talks a lot."

She replied, "She does? Oh, what the hell," she dismissed funnily. She drank her Fanta seemingly without a care in the world. We survived the emotional shift.

She then started to giggle. While she lay on her bed, I tried to feed her bites of a soft blueberry oatmeal cookie. She had issues, the last several weeks, with putting her tongue in the way of a bite—not sure whether to feel for the cup hole, consume a bite, suck a straw, or give a kiss. The movements would all get jumbled up in her reasoning. At this point, she stuck her tongue into the bite as I fed her a piece of this cookie. As such, she only bit a piece of the cookie, and the rest fell to her chest. I said, "Oops," and picked it up.

She laughed and said, "You're a kook."

I said, "I'm a kook?!? I'm kooky?!"

Oh, she got the giggles. "Yeah kooky," she said and laughed all the harder.

I got up to leave and told her I needed to do a bit more work for the day, and said, "But it's Friday. Yay Friday!!"

She replied back, "Oh!! Howl-yellow!!" Yes baby, Hallelujah! Hallelujah for wonderful moments and a chatty day.

AFTD Social Media Post – 5/27/19

WILLAMETTE NATIONAL CEMETERY

For the last twenty-two years, Maureen has honored her Uncle Johnny (SGT US Army) and Aunt Billie every single Memorial Day weekend since their passing. Theirs was a love story, and they died just eight days apart. They, and this annual remembrance with flowers, meant a lot to Maureen. So today I thought, I'll be damned if I let FTD rob her of that too. With the help of her wheelchair, we made our way to the grave site and placed a bouquet of mixed roses—their favorites. I never met a person with a bigger heart than Maureen. Best to you all.

Chapter 12

Dancing Differently

June started out rough. Maureen had stopped walking altogether, confined to the Geri chair and occasionally the wheelchair. She liked the comfort of the Geri chair—it was like a recliner on wheels. She dropped down to eighty-nine pounds and I think simply got too weak to walk. She could stand a bit if assisted.

She kept losing ground. Her physical rallies seemed like distant memories. She said very few words most of my visits. At night, in her pajamas and lying there but not asleep, I would notice her eyes partially open. The left one would often stay shut though, with the right one open like someone that had a stroke. She hardly responded. I held her hand and told her that I loved her.

She would nod and squeeze my hand, and on one of those nights came out of it and looked at me and said, "If you you you…don't try, you you can't keep him." She looked at me so lovingly as she said that. Given her propensity for swapping pronouns, I wondered if she kept clinging onto this world to stay with me.

She took the back of my hand and kissed it and looked at me again, "What is he?"

She had seen my tears. "Oh, I'm sad sometimes," I said. She looked concerned. "I just miss our fun times together."

"I know," she said. Did she? I wish I knew if she truly could recall all those times.

I reclined her bed, and she rolled over, and I lay up next to her back and gave her a light kiss.

"Is he go…blow blow…blowing my ear?" she asked.

"Yes," I replied.

"That's silly," she giggled and quickly fell asleep.

Afterward, I drove to the house—our home. I sat in the car to think about it all. In the house, everything was gone save for the few items in the garage: a mattress on the floor, a small table with two chairs, and some clothes in the closet. "Why won't this beautiful house sell?" I anguished in silence.

I squinted my eyes through tears as I thought of how frail Maureen had become. I kept trying my best. My best proved not good enough. I saw my baby slipping away. I saw her dying.

"Breathe," I thought. "Just breathe."

AFTD Social Media Post – 6/2/19

CHANGING PERSPECTIVES

"The question is not what you look at, but what you see." – Henry David Thoreau

My wife's perspective is changing (so must mine). FTD is a slow decline from what was to what things are now—only to change again as we blink. I have found her peripheral vision is gone. She uses her eyes less and hangs her head. In a reclined position or when she is fully rested, she looks up and smiles, and her eyes twinkle.

I think on my youth and Mr. Magoo—a delightful fellow with very poor eyesight that is always getting him into trouble. I am not sure who is more "Magoo", my wife or me. I think it is me. There are troublesome days where I look but do not always see.

She verbalizes so little these days, so I do my best. Questions like, "Would you like to eat some watermelon?" usually get no response. Sometimes the response is, "She thought he was there," or some other series of words with hidden meaning. Instead, I just try things and watch for the reaction.

I am still coaching the caregiving staff too. They tell her as they leave her room, "Your drink is on the table." You might as well tell her to jump on her unicorn. It is not going to happen.

You need to pick up her drink, take her hand, set the drink in her hand, close her fingers on it, and suggest she drink. If FTD allows, she probes for the drink hole with her tongue and will tip and drink. If not, any number of things can happen: she will just hold the cup indefinitely; she will compulsively turn the cup; she will turn it upside down; she will put her mouth to it and suck (not realizing she needs to tip it). We try straws, but often she bites down on the straw and will not suck on it or tries to put her tongue into the end of the straw. Sometimes she kisses the straw if I have not spaced my, "I love you" far enough away from my, "Please drink." The struggles are real. I think we are both Magoos.

She likes orange Fanta (I personally think it is ghastly). She drinks that from a bottle. She cannot do cans. She used to be able to twist the cap on and off but no longer. Small bottles are best, which are only sold in one grocery store every other fifth Thursday in odd numbered months (or so it seems).

As her eating declined, the doctor told us to choose calorie-dense foods. "Don't worry about healthy," he said. "Make every bite count." I stocked up on snacks in her room and brought milkshakes and ice cream. However, she was never a big eater, and she gained no weight. She is now down to 87.6 pounds but holding steady.

I have tried a new perspective and give her foods that I know she likes. She loves mandarin oranges. I cannot leave them in her room because she will bite them like an apple. I peel them and feed her one wedge at a time. She loves watermelon, so I feed her that too. In the last three weeks, she has eaten most of what I bring. These have so few calories, but she eats them.

I see things differently now and just give her what she likes. I have stopped worrying about whether she will ever put back on weight. I keep her comfortable.

I have also taken to sitting on the floor instead of beside her. Her head hangs low most of the time, and this helps with eye contact. I am literally changing MY perspective. I look up at her, and this often makes her smile and look back at me. I move from our Magoo vision to that familiar love.

Then staff sees someone on the floor and react like a code red. Nope not a fall, just an adapting husband.

The best thing we can do is change our perspective based on what we are experiencing. Keep it simple. She likes watermelon, so I try watermelon.

"Nobody said it'd be easy, they just promised it would be worth it." – Dr. Seuss

She is so worth it.

AFTD Social Media Post – 6/8/19

HER WORDS

"I have no idea why God made me the way that I am, but I am thankful he has brought such happiness and contentment to my life, and, of course, the laughter." – Maureen Patrick(-Rose) 1997 – in a letter to me two months after we started dating

My wife has the semantic variant of Primary Progressive Aphasia (svPPA). I do not know that it matters much anymore. They are just words now. Early on as we searched for answers and understanding, it mattered, so I read. I read a lot. I watched helplessly as the symptoms played out like in a textbook.

While it starts, and worsens, with words, the behavioral and mobility issues appear later as they are now. She uses a Geri chair most of the time now, especially in the afternoons and evenings when she is more tired and less mobile. Sometimes we get a few steps out of her in the mornings.

I mourn it all, but I think mostly I mourn the loss of her words.

In the past, she journaled a little, took a creative writing class, and wrote letters that I am pulling together now. We have inspirational cards that I used to leave by her mirror or stuck in her work bag. She saved them all, and they became her words to herself that she would read again and again for that encouragement. I once wrote on a small piece of paper left by the coffee pot "I love you banana bunches." She refused to put it away. It stayed by our coffee pot for years, so she owned those words too.

These few written words I will treasure, but I miss her spoken words most.

Her words were always caring, sweet, loving, encouraging, and heartfelt. However, in some of them, there were also tinges of sadness, self-doubt, and "still healing". She would be the first to admit she made a few mistakes before we met. I viewed them as her screaming out and nobody listening, but no matter what I said, her childhood trauma and struggles still shook her.

I approached our marriage trying to empower her. I did not want to change her words. They are hers. I wanted her to find more, new words, words of joy. She did, for more than twenty years, and I am happy for that.

FTD has now stolen most of those words back.

She cannot write. She cannot read much (maybe a word here or there). She has become more non-verbal each week, though there are still some words she uses, and we delight in those together.

There will be a loud sound in the next room, and it startles her. She looks at me and kind of smiles. She is searching for her words. "Crash Bang," I say. She giggles, "Yeah, Crash Bang." A phrase she has used for years.

When her grandkids were toddlers, she would sit and hold them and hear about their adventures and reply, "Holy cow!" They would laugh and she would change to "Holy chicken!" They would laugh harder and harder as she went through all the farm animals. I will say "Holy chicken" now, and she smiles.

For some reason, she had been hooked for years on the Finding Nemo scene of the seagulls shouting, "Mine. Mine.

Mine." She mimicked it every time and giggled with the grandkids. I hear it in my head still.

My goals are simple:

Keep her comfortable (happy where I can). Keep her words, and all that she is and was. I tell myself, "Don't let them fade from memory."

"Could it be I will disappear, having lasted not much longer then the pearls of dew that barely cling to the lotus leaves?" – Murasaki Shikibu, The Tale of Genji

---

That June marked three years since her diagnosis. The FTD had robbed so much from her in that time, including her words. She still had them in her mind, but the link between her mind and her mouth got broken, as did the link between her mind and the rest of her body. She had so much trouble making herself do anything anymore. Sometimes she would do things and think she had done something else. Sometimes I think she just knew she could not make herself do as she wanted and got sad.

I really saw that manifest itself in June: she had become very unhappy. I got her out in the sun as much as possible, often in one of the chairs. Sometimes I would roll the Geri chair right out the front door of the care facility and roll her to a nearby park on campus or take a long roll around the block. Some days she would act like she enjoyed it and others she was seemingly lost in thought. I do not know if she was remembering the days that she could walk it or thinking about something else entirely. Could she comprehend all that she no longer could do?

I still took her on outings a couple of times each week. For those, we used the collapsible wheelchair. I would lift her into the front seat and buckle her in, and sometimes I'd get a pat on my head.

Often, she would see the red box of Altoids and launch for those. Sometimes we stayed in the car at a park with the windows rolled down so she felt the breeze on her face, and other times we got out and rolled through the park together. I would gauge her mood. If she seemed receptive, we took longer outings to the rose gardens. Again, she took in some of it, but generally seemed saddened.

I tried to stay positive for her and did so most of the time. But when she would not eat or not speak, just glance at me as I came in, or just stared off rather than react, those moments broke my heart.

One night as she was lying in bed just after getting her pajamas on, she remained completely silent and had done so for the whole evening. She offered no reciprocal language to any of mine. I rested my head on her chest sadly and stroked her arm. That night, she raised her hand and stroked my hair. I let her. She spoke, "You are loved." I turned and smiled at her. She looked right at me and said again, "You are loved."

FTD sometimes does this. It lets you borrow back words for a moment, only to steal them back again. She said nothing the rest of the night.

I would get very few words in a day's time and sometimes, many times, simply no response, just stares off and away. "What is she thinking?" I wondered. We still had our connection. Often, though, she kept her eyes closed. I would lean down and whisper in her ear, "I love you." She would just smile, eyes closed—good enough for me.

I shared the recent developments with her daughter and son by text (the only way they communicated) every couple of weeks. I asked if they had any questions, as I typically did. A day later her son would text, "Thanks for the update," but her daughter rarely responded.

Without their input or, of course, that of Maureen herself, I often felt lost. I tried things—some worked, some did not. I would try them again the next day or week and find that those that did not work before, suddenly did and vice versa. I bounced ideas off the AFTD support group and listened to other ideas that worked for them.

For those cared for and caregivers alike, we find it heartbreaking, confusing, frustrating, maddening, hopeless, and nerve-wracking. But we can also find uplifting, joyous, hysterical, tender, and heart-warming moments. Me feeding a cup of soup to my wife one afternoon could frustrate or delight me. She could not always open her mouth when I asked her to. My heart broke watching her waste away. I also, though, embraced tender joy at her figuring out after several attempts how to open her mouth and take that bite. I said, "Good job baby. That was perfect," and she grinned. While hard, each day I tried again to spin it in my head and heart (not always succeeding). I kept thinking "Celebrate the magnificence of the ordinary." Even the smallest accomplishments are huge.

I love you baby. I just wander through life right now trying to do the right things for you. For me, I have no idea what that is.

AFTD Social Media Post – 6/15/19

CHERISH

How can I list every cherished moment with my wife since we first started dating on December 28, 1996? I shall not even try. Part of what we cherish is the intimacy of the memory.

John Pavlovitz wrote an essay regarding the loss of a very dear loved one. He says, "You lose the part of you that only they knew. You lose some of your story."

Yes, so true. There are many parts of my life only she knows, that only she has experienced, and vice versa. I thought on this today and had a hard time leaving from our time together. With each day, it seems so apparent to me that the days remaining are so very few.

Her facility director randomly said to me yesterday, "Maureen is a strong woman." Caught off guard, all I could say was, "Yes. Yes, she is."

Maureen does seem like she is holding on—for what I do not know. Is she afraid? Confused? Does she want to tell me (or someone else) something? Is she waiting for me to tell HER something? To see someone once more? One would think as we near the end, the questions would fade—they do not.

I rolled her out to the courtyard today under the shade of a gazebo. She was grinning, as I had just told her, "I love you with all my heart." The reciprocal language has been gone a few weeks now, but this grin tells me she heard me, and it registered. That is all I need.

The painful thing with Maureen's FTD/cancer combo is the "dying" over and over again. Based on the words of doctors, nurses, hospice, and caregivers, I have buried her many times and sobbed holding her hand by her bed so much.

She has lived on and provided me more precious memories, but my life has been zombie-like for months. Not knowing what to do, I keep holding on. She processes, and says, almost nothing, but enough that she is still elated most times when I come into the room. I do a "Ta-da!", so even if she does not look up, she smiles.

Parts of me have died, are dying, die again and again, but I would not trade this extra time with her for anything. It dawned on me though that I HAVE traded it. I traded it for feelings of sadness, loss, pre-grief, and staring at the inevitable. While each day I DO struggle to find the positive and to celebrate the magnificence of the ordinary, I still get down my fair share of the time too. I need to instead cherish even more this extra time with her.

I had an improv teacher years ago. He gave us great advice the first day of class, "When you come here, make yourself completely available. Whatever baggage you brought with you—troubles with relationships, money, work, etc.—leave them at the door. There is nothing that you can do to fix them in the next ninety minutes, so just set them down and commit to our time together. When we're done, that baggage that you set down will still be there for you to pick back up, but for a short time, you allowed yourself the freedom to be immersed in the moment."

I encourage you all to do the same. If you are focusing on the bad, the inevitable, the overwhelming—please stop it. There are only so many moments to cherish with your loved one, and who really wants to miss one of those?

As I said, Maureen had become more and more non-verbal. That works to your disadvantage in a care facility, as the limited resources often default to the easy fixes.

One day, I arrived just after lunch and they had her sat at a table alone in her Geri chair with nobody to engage her. She had some food and drink in front of her. She looked flushed in her cheeks. I saw her lips still and parted like when she had not drunk anything in some time. She also looked out of sorts with her hands running over and over again along her hair bringing it down across her eyes.

As I entered and gave my "Ta-Da", she looked up and said, "You're a liar." Uh-oh. She had not spoken much those days—not a good start.

"I should...you...go," she stammered out. I found out the staff had just changed her before bringing her to the table, and she did not like them fussing with her. Who does really?

I held her hand and whispered in her ear, "I think you are beautiful." She then did something she had not done in probably two years. She looked at me, smiled, and batted her eyes. Men, you know what I speak of: when a lady gives you a look and then flutters her eyelids and you melt into a puddle of goo and will do anything for her.

Anyway, her mood shifted to a more positive one then. FTD moods can change on a dime. I still had to read her body language for the eating and drinking, as she had not yet decided that she wanted to. Rather than verbalizing it, she pushed food away with pursed lips when she did not want to eat. I knew better with FTD to not force it. After better than an hour of negotiating, though, we got enough food and drink in her.

A guest came in to play the piano, and a few residents gathered to hear his music. I had a caregiver help her to a spot with the group to listen.

I left but returned about 6 o'clock. They had Maureen in the big room in front of the TV with some old movie playing that was twenty years too old for her—something from the classic big band era. She paid no attention to it at all, just staring off and nobody engaging her. Again, with limited care resources and her inability to verbalize what she wanted, they chose the simple path.

I rolled her in her Geri chair down the hall to a quieter spot by one of the couches. Not knowing how long she had sat in the chair, I lifted her out, carrying and cradling her in my arms for a few moments. She leaned into me.

I reminded myself at that moment, "Never easy, but always worth it."

I said I would never stop dancing with my wife. She could not walk anymore, but this rocking in my arms worked nearly as well.

Initially, when we transferred her from her Geri chair to her bed and vice versa, she would panic and say "No"—doubting her ability to stand. Despite softly talking to her and physically supporting her every second, she would still get nervous.

Again, I said I would never stop dancing with my wife. I cradled her as we transferred. She did not panic. She nestled her head against my neck. I swayed her to one of her songs playing on the phone in my pocket:

> "Wouldn't it be nice if we could wake up
> In the morning when the day is new?
> And after having spent the day together
> Hold each other close the whole night through?
>
> Happy times together we've been spending
> I wish that every kiss was never ending
> Oh, wouldn't it be nice?"
>
> – Beach Boys

Eventually I placed her on the adjacent couch, and we visited for a time. I say visited in that I spoke to her, and she gave me occasional "Mm-hmms" or "Yeahs".

A couple of lost gentlemen were wandering back and forth near us, speaking loudly. When I tried to help them, it threw Maureen off. She heard my voice and thought I had spoken to her. She did not know how to respond.

After a few minutes of this (and the men now arguing with each other), I thought her room would work best. I flagged a caregiver down for the men. I rolled my lovely wife back to her room and got her to stand as I held her. She stood a bit using her own strength, but eventually wanted to sit on the bed.

I then swung her feet up and picked her up to get her further up the bed. She did not resist it as much as she used to and sometimes, as I said, even leaned in. I explained what I planned to do as I did it, and I think the repetition helped.

I lay her down and played a music box I bought for her at Pittock Mansion the day before. She rested—only occasionally opening her eyes. She spoke a little, so I stopped the music, trying to catch the words. She spoke soft words, and she always looked so tired those days. She opened her eyes and stared right at me. I put the backs of a couple of fingers against her right cheek, and she leaned her head into them, let her eyes close, and said, "...so thankful for you." That soft and low voice spoke words as clear as before all this FTD started—she just sounded tired now. Wow! Nothing will melt your heart quicker.

She spoke those four words on my fifty-second birthday. To this day, the best gift that I ever received.

We are the same hopelessly devoted couple from three years ago, just living a life with rougher edges.

On the later visits that summer when I would bring her mother, Maureen sort of recognized her mom but not too much. Her mother shared a few stories from their past with Maureen, hoping to spark some response, but with none, she shifted to her own daily activities, which garnered, of course, no response either.

We tried getting food or drink in Maureen beyond just during mealtimes, so the staff handed me a small bowl of pineapple while we visited. She remained mostly quiet, only speaking a few words here and there. I then asked for a simple turkey sandwich, but she only took a few bites of that—no longer interested. She drank plenty, including her Ensure. During all this, her mother just watched or stared off out the window.

Maureen got sleepy, so after about ninety minutes I flagged down a staff person and took her mother back to her apartment. I think she saw the same things I did; she saw Maureen fading. She asked what arrangements I had made. I told her of the niche at Rest-Haven in Eugene that I had secured for her and I. I mentioned the legacy memorial I had started coordinating at Pittock Mansion.

Oddly, she asked if I planned on having a service. I am sure I did not hide my shock at that question well. I said, "Yes, of course there will be, but I have not made any arrangements as yet, because her condition has been imminent for six months now."

"Well, I would get that all lined up. What town will it be in?" she asked.

"I imagine up here in Portland, as this is her home. I have pulled together a few things, but actual arrangements won't happen 'till after her passing." I tried not to mimic her clinical nature, but she wanted the facts.

She continued, "Well, it could just be putting her ashes somewhere and not be a big service. She lived as long in Redmond or Eugene."

I told her I planned to have a larger, formal service. I also said I would pre-write memorial statements and place obituaries in papers in Weiser, Idaho and also in Oregon in Redmond, Eugene, and Portland.

This seemed to satisfy her. I understood her desire to have things in place, but I also refused to rush to bury my wife. I wanted to enjoy the time we had left. We all grieve differently. I had to keep reminding myself of that.

She had already, in her mind, buried her daughter. She preferred not to think of Maureen in the present, but as she had lived, perhaps even how she had lived as a child. She made the comment to me regarding an ex-wife of her husband's son as her "substitute daughter now." I left myself no tongue that day. I bit it clean off rather than share my hurt and anger at that statement with Maureen still very much alive.

Perhaps, I considered, Maureen and I had become the only ones still hanging on.

Caitlin, her hospice manager, called me that next day and said she had grown more concerned by how tired Maureen had become and the ongoing lack of appetite. She used the phrase that "organs could start shutting down." I told her I understood. She reiterated that she still considered her comfort critical but that we had no plan to prolong her life or cure anything. She had told me this six months earlier. I teared up a bit over the phone. Caitlin said the staff talk about me and my devotion and tenderness toward Maureen. I thanked her and wanted to tell her that I felt so incredibly inadequate but instead said nothing.

This had become so very real. Mornings had reduced to just eating and drinking and changing. Afternoons I focused on getting her sun and trying for some joy. In the evenings, I routinely sat and held her hand and would get a few words, but she always drifted in and out of sleep. She winced but not about her wounds. Her bottom hurt from sitting so long and having no padding left on her rear from the weight loss. I would roll her over and tuck a pillow behind her to keep her on her side. That seemed to help.

Evenings had almost no words except when they messed with her to do her bandage and get her pajamas on. Those words generally broke down to just kind of negative sounds and the occasional no. She really seemed to not fully wake up though—like talking in her sleep. We lay her on her back with her head slightly elevated. They would roll her throughout the night to relieve pressure on joints.

A couple of evenings, I worried whether she would make it through the night. I asked the head nurse Mary if she thought it looked imminent and if I needed to camp out there. While always hard to tell, she did not think so each of those times.

I did not sleep much those evenings, so I should have just stayed anyway. I lay in bed worried I would get a call in the middle of the night or in the morning to tell me that she had passed. Those calls never came. I loved her so much (love her still) and wanted the best for her whatever that "best" might have meant.

My poor baby. Life has treated you so poorly.

By the end of June, Maureen could no longer walk or stand. I could stand her up while hugging her for a few moments. This would relieve all the tension on her joints. I would gently sway-dance with her, rocking her body to one of our songs. Her arms would not make it all the way around my neck but would lift to both my arms tenderly. She seemed to like it. She hummed. She then needed to sit back down on the bed. I made these our personal bed-to-chair or chair-to-bed transfers.

Some nights, not sleeping, I would come by around midnight just to watch her sleep. A different kind of staff works the graveyard shift. They provide much less care, since most residents do sleep through the night. Unless the nurse directs a check-in frequency on the charts, it rarely happens from what I've observed. Once, a caregiver accidentally put Maureen's air unit on heat rather than cool, and a medium fan, so I happened upon a blast furnace in the room. I just shook my head. I switched it to AC and down to a low fan and stripped all but the sheet off. She stirred a lot as though uncomfortable, so I went to give her water, but they had left the cup on her nightstand empty. I got her some fresh water. "Clods," I thought.

They changed her bandage twice a day, in the morning and evening. Both wounds of course remained—the cancerous cells kept them from ever healing. They would change from oozing a little to oozing a lot and clear to a yellowish substance. Other than getting messed with for the clean bandages, she did not seem to mind the wounds themselves. They managed the pain well, and she no longer rubbed at them, so they stopped using the onesies late spring. She left the bandages alone now. They had become part of her routine.

Some days she would surprise me. She would just be alert and looking around, acting as if she had rallied. I used to get excited and then let down when she had a relapse. I needed to stop succumbing to those rollercoasters and just enjoy the good moments, as I preached to others.

On those alert days, I would come around the corner and she would say, "My my my husband. Oh, I just love love love you." That just melted my heart, as she had not called me her husband in several weeks. On those mornings, we could sit together and have breakfast consisting of fruit, eggs, and her chocolate drink (Ensure) as we called it in her white plastic Starbucks cup. It seemed really good. Other days, her alert state came later in the afternoon. She ate best at those times.

Sometimes she would eat but keep her eyes closed. It seemed to work by smell. I would bring up watermelon, cantaloupe, and honey dew to her mouth, and she would slightly smell it and open her mouth to eat it. With a broccoli and potato dish they made, I would do the same, but she smelled it and kept her mouth closed and said no. Her nose still worked well.

She did not like anything that took much time to chew. She held food in her cheeks, like she forgot to swallow. Soft and slippery food slid down her throat easily. I always worried about it going down the wrong pipe; FTD has a very real threat of aspiration pneumonia. One day, as I fed her, she choked just a bit, and my heart jumped into my throat. What had I done? It happened with tiny mandarin oranges. It seemed to clear on its own without any assistance. I watched her for several minutes after. It passed, and I sighed in relief. Would she need to move to pureed foods?

I let the nurses know multiple times that she held her food and would forget to swallow. Perhaps her childhood phobia of choking had kicked in. I never knew. Sadly, unless I brought something, they fed her the same food they fed the rest of the residents.

She still drank pretty well. She used a straw about 90% of the time. Sometimes though, she would bite the straw or just put it in her mouth and forget to suck on it. I would take them out of her mouth and try again in a minute to see if I could catch her mind on the right track. That "reset" seemed to work most of the time.

When I caught her just right, she would grab a glass or the plastic bottle and drink directly from that. However, one time, I noticed she drove a crease into the bridge of her nose because she kept tipping the glass to get the water but did not tip her head. Wires had crossed again. When I helped her, she would often think I was trying to take something from her, so she fought it. We did a lot of negotiating.

She struggled with utensils—both to use and to receive in her mouth. As such, I handfed her a lot, using my finger to put the food in her mouth. However, when I spoon-fed her a mini-blizzard, she would gobble that thing right down.

Still, though, she never gained any weight and continued to lose more and more.

AFTD Social Media Post – 7/1/19

MY WISP

"Someone frail, slight, or fleeting."

I have seen a lot of things in my life—more than most. As such, little shakes me.

While I look at my wife, I see a beautiful woman. I also see someone inexorably wasting away, struggling to keep finding that joy and optimism that she was known for her whole life.

I entered her room today, and she was half-sleeping with slow and shallow breathing through her nose. I said it was her husband, and with her eyes still closed, she grinned.

I held her hand 'till she rousted herself—a few seconds or several minutes, I do not know or care.

She moved from her side to her back and widened her eyes. Each time, she takes in the room and stops on me, studying. I ask her if she wants water. Nothing. I ask again softly. "Mm-hmm."

A glass with a lid and flexible straw is on her nightstand, and I take it to her mouth to drink. She bites on the straw and leaves lips parted. I ask her to close her lips and suck. I can see at that moment in her processing I might as well have asked her to rebuild an engine.

I pull the straw out and suggest we try using just the cup and tip it gently to her mouth, and she sips. Again, we try, and some spills, and I am quick to dab it. She does not want that method again, so we go back to the straw. This time, she takes to it and drinks fully. Such are our days—processes and perceptions blowing like wisps of grass.

They have her in bed in just a T-shirt. It accentuates how frail, slight, fleeting she is. She is still my wife and the love of my life, but just about 80 pounds left.

She looks at me more intently. "My...husband." She smiles as I tear up. I hold her hand, and she continues to smile. Just as quickly, that rare smile fades.

I am kneeling on the floor next to her bed and continue to gently cry. Dylan sings "Make you feel my love" as she reaches her tiny arm to my cheek. She says nothing but her touch says volumes. We look at each other for a few seconds or several minutes, I do not know or care.

We hold hands, my wisp and me. That was tonight and how I spend most of my nights. What a joy and treasure.

"Everybody born comes from the Creator as trailing wisps of glory." – Maya Angelou

---

Again, she did not use many words anymore. The staff told me that week that as they were feeding her breakfast, she said "murder" to one of them. They did not know where that came from. She could not choose words much anymore. She tended to clump words as a cluster of positive and a cluster of negative, and then pull out a random word for "yes" when she liked something or "no" when she did not. When she said "murder", she meant, "No I do not want that breakfast food."

Sadly, most of her words became increasingly harder to understand. Even a single word then often sounded like gibberish—a combination of random consonants and a stuttered repetition.

She also spoke softly. I could hardly pick out a word anymore to repeat as I had done in the past. I did that to cope with her changed language and give her affirmative responses. She thought she said something that I should understand, so now that I could no longer understand, she became frustrated. That may have led to the increased silence.

The weeks in July passed with a blur. One day blended into the next—one week into the next. I waited. For what, I did not know. I sat there afraid to take a step too far one way or the other for fear of losing Maureen. I perhaps waited in some aspect of my mind to suddenly discover that Maureen did not have FTD, that this had all been a cruel joke or imbalance and that she would just wake up one day and be fine, or at least on the mend.

I fooled myself with this thinking when I saw a glimmer in her eyes—even for an instant. I desperately wanted her rallies to turn to reversals.

I would start tracking the positives. She called me husband once in the first two weeks of July. She said she loved me twice—though both times I asked her, and she said "yes" or "mmm-hmm". I took it. She smiled half a dozen times. I relished these scarce moments.

I would take her out for a drive or to the Portland Memory Garden in the sun, with a slight breeze and the smell of flowers in raised beds, so she could touch and smell them from her wheelchair. She smiled, and with guidance, smelled the summer blooms. We made that trip a few times. I took to packing the wheelchair in the backseat all the time, even if we did not plan to get out.

On those outings, she might stay silent or might get a bit more talkative. Still not making much sense, she would just offer bits and pieces and generally spoke softly. The pace of her speech slowed. She would speak for a moment, and then fade out again. She just went in and out.

Sometimes the words, while soft, would make sense. For instance, when I picked her up from the chair to transfer her, she no longer struggled and sometimes added, "You...so good." I took it as a win.

As she seemed frail but stable, I ventured a beach trip with her. She loved the beach this time of year.

AFTD Social Media Post – 7/19/19

GIGGLING

I love to watch my wife in a fit of giggles. She has a delightful sense of humor, and a soft spot for bodily functions gone awry. Mr. Creosote in The Meaning of Life left her in stitches. She also howled at the Blazing Saddles campfire scene and Leslie Neilson leaving his lapel mic on in the bathroom in The Naked Gun.

My wife has not giggled in a long time and did not today. I, however, AM laughing at the absurdity of what transpired.

I had planned to take Maureen to the Oregon Coast today (ninety minutes away) for a single overnight. She was in decent spirits. I had the wheelchair, the meds, her current necessities, etc. I thought, "There is nothing I have not planned for." Oh, how wrong I was.

We are fifteen miles from the facility, going down the highway and she starts to uh...well...expel. Oddly, my impulse was to cup my hand near her mouth. I guess I thought my hand was the size of a catcher's mitt. It is not. I am now driving fifty miles an hour with one hand on the wheel and the other covered in vomit.

She understood she got sick, but the apathy kicked in, and there was no trying to contain it. She just let it fly. She sat there listening to the music.

The next off-ramp is a mile down the freeway. When you have puke in your hand, sixty seconds seems like an eternity.

The exit is the Oregon Zoo. I had to laugh, "We were going to the beach, not the zoo." I parked and began clean-up. There had been a blanket on her lap, and she was wearing a tunic over a T-shirt. I stripped off the tunic and balled it in the saturated blanket. A little more clean up, and I thought, "Perhaps she will be fine the rest of the way." No.

Twenty miles later—the second round of liquid projectiles. I go to catch it again. What am I thinking?!? I am now scrambling for a turnoff again and find a rural road off the highway. Again, I had one hand steering and the other dripping.

I think, "Skip the beach." There is no blanket, and her pants and T-shirt are now saturated. With every attempt to maintain her dignity, I discreetly changed her top and bottoms on the far side of this, thankfully, deserted road. Down to seventy-eight pounds, she cannot stand, walk, etc., so it's dead weight that I am trying to lift, wrestle, and keep covered. We will not speak of the growing smell.

I am now travelling back to her facility on the highway over a bridge when we have event number three. "God?! Message received! I already turned around!" Of course, I reacted with my right hand again, as though there is some broken chip in my head. This time, it is running off her shirt and onto the seat. I wipe my hand on my pants and reach behind me to find ANYthing. I feel a package of napkins on the floor that I brought for potential messes: this qualifies. Tearing them open with my teeth, I grab handfuls and shove them between her hip and the seat to sop up the spill like applying a tourniquet to a wound.

There is nowhere to turn off. I am on a BRIDGE! One hand steering and the other wiping with wads of napkins. All the while, I am asking my dear wife if she is ok and trying to wipe her mouth and give her water.

I would turn off in a mile and find some way to change her top, but only five miles from the facility, so I think, just get her back, and clean it up there.

Two miles to go, and the fourth and final episode occurs. As I have brought my hand up to catch it three times, why not this last? I have a few remaining napkins in my hand— most are soiled on the floor mat between my legs.

At the facility, we get her cleaned up, changed, and in her bed. She was fine. She looked at me and grinned. I said that I was sorry we did not make it to the beach. I placed my fingers (washed) against her cheek, and she leaned into them. We are keeping her hydrated tonight to replenish what she lost, and she is resting peacefully.

Her cancer causes pain near her stomach. Her weight loss causes pain due to no "padding". As such, hospice has had her on a hydromorphone painkiller called Dilaudid. According to them (on a call I made tonight), a potential side effect is motion sickness. Really?!?!? They suggested a patch behind her ear next time.

FTD is quite the experience, and I am thankful the love of my life is well. Yes, I still call her that, despite today's resemblance to Mr. Creosote. She would have giggled.

You have to have a strong stomach and a lot of patience for FTD. Messes WILL happen, and in those advanced conditions your loved ones often simply do not understand all the fuss.

Late July, after grabbing a bit of dinner, I returned to her facility to make sure they had her sleeping, comfortable, etc. In the dark room, I came to her bedside and peered closely to find feces all over her face, hand, blankets, etc. She had apparently messed her pants, got uncomfortable, reached in to scratch, and did not realize she had gotten feces on her hand and then everywhere else as she slumbered.

I called the team in, and together we got her stripped, the bed stripped, her cleaned, new pajamas and bedding, etc. We got her back to square one. I did not blame the care staff. It just happened, probably between her hourly checks. In the dark, they just do a glance. Nobody gave her as many looks and attention as I did. I knew that.

Maureen only got agitated by us rushing around.

If you find yourself in a caregiving role, you should prepare. Your loved one might also momentarily, and inadvertently, turn on you.

I fed Maureen dinner and tried to get her to eat some broccoli. I normally handfed her most food as she seemed to take it better. She did not want the broccoli, but I wanted her to eat something other than just fruit. I persisted and finally got the broccoli into her mouth. Slow to pull my finger out, she looked right at me and bit as hard as she could. I screamed in that grand room; it hurt a lot. I think my scream startled her as much as others around us. It took all my concentration (and a three count) to just say, "Honey. That really hurt." She gave me a one-word reply, "No." Message received.

I never stopped loving her unconditionally.

AFTD Social Media Post – 8/2/19

BEAUTIFULLY NORMAL

Yes, my wife has FTD. Yes, my wife has lost a dangerous amount of weight. Yes, she is often non-verbal, totally dependent, and terminal, but those things are not her. They do not define her.

Her soul, and the souls and experiences of each of our loved ones are what define them.

It makes us angry. It makes us confused. It makes us sad. It, it, it...FTD, not our loved ones. This organization is AFTD, not ALO.

I encourage us caregivers to try stripping away the FTD from our loved ones for a moment. I know it is hard because it hits us in the face all the time but look at them—the real them. Are they, behind the FTD, still our loved one, still beautiful, still normal?

My wife bit her lip bad this week because her brain is not telling her how to make her muscles do what they should. How many of us have ever bit our lip?

My wife would not respond and kept to herself the following day, likely hurting. How many of us retreat when we are hurting?

My wife only eats fruit and sweet things now and bit my finger when I tried to feed her broccoli. How many of us have foods we crave or don't want?

When a pleasant sound, sight, or smell catches her notice, she innocently and silently smiles. How many of us have been touched by a memory triggered by our senses?

She cannot walk, shower, change, or use the toilet without full assistance. How many of us have ever felt weak or needed help with something and leaned on a loved one?

My wife no longer has the capacity or fortitude to do all the travel, concerts, eating out, or other fun things we once did. How many of us have some obstacle keeping us from doing what we want?

She is often tired and has a small window each day where she is verbal, but then dozes off. How many of us have ever felt drained, tired, or simply didn't want to do anything?

She was lucid for a few moments yesterday (has not been that way in months) and said she was scared and did not want to die. How many of us have had something that terrified us?

How is she, or YOUR loved one, not still both unique and just like us?

I am neither naïve nor wearing rose colored glasses. I too live with the financial, emotional, and physical pressures. I know the reality of what is happening and will continue to happen. Yes, I weep knowing she is going to die.

I will die someday too.

As will you.

Our loved ones are each so unique—each with souls.

Just like us, they too are beautifully normal.

Among the challenges for Maureen, our personal financial story looked no better. The house had sat on the market for a year and did not sell. We received a single offer literally the day the realtor's contract expired. The buyer offered something ridiculously low, so I had to reject it. Even though financial resources continued to dwindle, rather than renewing her contract, I took it off the market with the intent to relist in the spring.

I still just used the one bedroom but had gotten tired of the uncertainty. I decided one thing in my life needed stability. I spent that first August weekend moving our now limited number of things out of the garage and spread them back into the house. I decided to start living in our home again. The mattress on the floor and occasional parceling through garage boxes had gotten old.

This simple shift made me feel better. Perhaps that improved attitude rubbed off on Maureen. While she had remained quiet for some time, she had yet another rally—what a treat. However, I also thought, "How many rallies does she get?"

She became chatty, smiling, and very pleasant. She even had some moments when she really looked at me and seemed to understand her situation. Perhaps it frightened her if she popped out of her state even for a moment. That could scare someone—to see what their life had transformed into. For now, though, she stayed happy and talkative.

I had her in her Geri chair in the courtyard. We sat close, holding hands. I gave her some flirty banter, "Hubba hubba."

She chuckled and softly said, "Shit."

I responded, "Shit?! Did you just say shit?!"

She chuckled again, "Pretty much." She drank her soda with a silly grin—priceless.

Now mid-August, I thought of the ups and downs in that one year since I first placed her in the care facility. I could not help but look back and wonder whether I had done the right thing.

Many advised me that I had waited too long. "Too long?!" I would question. "How exactly was it too long?"

They would quip, "Well, she was a good candidate many months ago."

Oh really?! That is the timing huh?! She "qualifies", so out the door with a boot in the ass?!

I know they did not mean it that way. However, until they had walked in our shoes, they could not understand our life together— our hearts. They did not understand that I bucked hard against it, that I fought it 'till the last hour, that I kept weaving and dodging to find a way to make it work at home or at an alternate facility where we could still live together or with in-home care or, or, or...

They did not hear my screams at God that day a year ago when I placed her there and walked out. They did not see the tears that flowed for days and still flow now a year later. They did not feel the guilt that I have felt every day since. I shot a self-inflicted hole in my heart.

However, a year later, I knew I had made the right decision. I wished differently but knew better.

I would offer these tips for others contemplating placing their loved ones into a care facility:

1. Thorough research for the right facility pays off. It impacts everyone if you have to change facilities later.

2. Understand all the costs upfront and when/if those might change.

3. Make a list of as many questions about their care and services as you can think of and ask all your questions.

4. Provide a write-up of your loved one's life, including their likes and dislikes.

5. Visit often but call others to visit too.

6. You are not to blame for what does or does not happen there, but if you see something that you do not like, speak up. You are their advocate. Insist on positive changes.

7. This decision helps you to provide better care for them too, because it gives you physical and emotional rest.

8. Your caregiving does not stop because they live in a care facility. You will still be involved in their care.

9. Take them on outings or arrange for such. They will always still crave the outdoors, stimulation, and inter-action whether they show it or not.

My reflection brought to light some truths for Maureen and I. She had started spiraling over two years prior. Placing her in the facility had not hastened, or slowed, that descent. When I had to work, I knew they would keep her safe, yet I still got to see her as much as I wanted or could and did with her as much as I wanted or could. FTD became the limiting factor, not the facility. Despite having a job, I still saw her every day, two to three times a day. As such, we made several wonderful memories in that last year with holidays, outings, and quiet times. Those wonderful memories had pain, but also laughter and love.

Friends and family generally kept distant, though some did visit occasionally. People just behave within their nature, and I had to accept that. She and I travelled much of this journey alone. Many people still cared very much for her, but infinitely less than I did. I had to accept that too.

I know the staff there tried hard, even if they still remained generally naïve about FTD. I kept trying to coach them. I reminded myself that these good and compassionate people still tried to find ways to help residents celebrate life.

They decorated for holidays and had special brunches and even held an annual carnival and an annual luau in the main room. For the luau they had decorations, and music, and virgin mai tais and pina coladas. They had a Hawaiian dancing trio of ladies, spirited food of pulled pork, sticky rice, and more, and enough room for everyone who wanted to come.

I brought one of Maureen's dresses from our Hawaii and Mexico trips plus her summer wedges (though she remained in her Geri chair) and a pair of her Hawaiian-made earrings. With her frail nature, I supplemented the dress with a long-sleeved shirt to keep her warm. She looked beautiful and handled the activity surprising well, given her normal aversion to crowds.

I had come to learn over the prior year that although I had planned a very different outcome for our marriage and knew she would want a different path for her life if she could express it, we could still make it work. We could still create good memories and still love each other and spend time together.

Those memories sustain me now. The end came soon after.

Chapter 13

Our Last Dance

Maureen's confusion increased. While I still got the occasional gleeful, "It's my husband!", which I treasured each and every time, I could also see a breakdown of even basic understanding. She started tasting and licking her skin and pajamas.

She had returned to some oral exploratory activity. I warned staff that we had to keep small inedibles away from Maureen 'till this passed. She really liked to hold things. She liked to clutch small things as part of having control. I thought blankets and clothes wouldn't hurt, but I did a sweep through her room and removed everything that could fit in her mouth or could even break off in her mouth.

While doing so, I found the old metal handwarmer in a flowered Coach purse I had left for her in her room. It measured about six inches long and was slightly smaller than a cell phone. She could not swallow something that big, but she almost immediately put it in her mouth when I handed it to her. I had to take it away, fearing she might bite down hard on it and break something off. I had no idea why this tendency developed again after so long.

Not a lot else changed initially.

I loved (and love) Maureen so deeply. I had no idea what the future held, or I denied it to myself. I rocked her as I transferred her from chair to bed. We dance-swayed to another one of her songs, and she tucked in against me again, burying her head. She said nothing.

We captured a few more tender moments that summer.

AFTD Social Media Post – 8/17/19

A GOOFY KIND OF LOVE

On the fiftieth anniversary of the greatest music/love festival of all time, I thought I might reflect on how music has kept our love alive despite FTD.

When we are desperate, when the chips are down, we will try anything to survive. I will be honest; I am starting to feel a little worried as I watch things progress with my lovely bride. So much so, that today I tried something rash...I serenaded her.

Yes, despite her FTD, she gave me a shocked look. I cannot say I blame her. I sound like a cowbell drug down a gravel road. It is not pretty.

In the high school musicals, the choral director would hear me and I think internally wept at the horror of my voice. I remember Mr. Anderson taking me aside and asking if I could just do my best to blend in with the chorus and sing quieter.

I love music but have no musical talent, yet my wife is still my biggest fan.

My wife loves music, and she has talent. She played the saxophone in her high school marching band. Later in life, despite her shyness, she joined a women's choir. As a retirement gift, I got her piano lessons for four years 'till the FTD became too intense. Her uncle made her a Celtic harp, and she played her way through that. She has a great ear, so imagine her pain at my drunken cat warbling.

Nowadays, she listens to a CD player I have set in her room or a playlist on my iPhone of thirty or so of her favorite songs on shuffle (no earphones, as those bother her). Most tunes are older, but a few more contemporary. Some have emotional meaning, like our first date song or one from our honeymoon, and others are just fond memories she can still hum to. She rarely attempts the words anymore. When I "sing" the words to try and prompt her, her humming stops, and she listens to me—probably perplexed by that sound of breaking glass amongst the dog howls.

She had the great fortune of going to see Elvis Presley live in 1976. Since we have been together, I have made it one of my missions to take her to as many theatrical musicals, music festivals, and concerts as I could. This included some of the absolute classics. Our favorite concerts were with the Rolling Stones and Paul McCartney.

Music has been such an integral part of our marriage, as it is now, as she battles the end of FTD. If she is having a bad day, not talking much, not responding, showing anxious or angry behavior, I will play the music for her, and it relaxes her. This is not just background noise (like leaving the TV on), as that has the opposite effect. This is HER music and shuffled, so she is listening for the next song. We dance best we can these days even if just cradled in my arms.

I am surprised that with thirty-five other residents in her facility, I never hear a radio played out of any of their rooms and never in any of the sitting rooms. There is a radio in the grand room, but I only hear it on a few days per week and only briefly, maybe an hour.

There Maureen and I are, with the iPhone playing in her lap as I roll her down the halls or in the courtyard. We just enjoy the tunes, humming along and stopping to look at each other. I mine her for her remaining smiles. Yes, we will do anything to keep our goofy love alive a little longer.

AFTD Social Media Post – 8/24/19

HAPPY HEART

If I live to be a hundred, I still do not think I will fully understand FTD.

As I have posted, my wife is steadily declining and perhaps near the end. Most days, she says very little, and it is typically jumbled. Her eyes are always down. She eats almost nothing and cannot walk anymore. She even seems a bit depressed lately.

I have been feeling like she is in a rut and needs something a little special, though I understand the importance of routine. I planned to take her to our old house (not yet sold) for dinner, a fire on the deck, and an overnight stay.

All preparations made, and I pick her up about 2:30 this afternoon. She is in decent spirits, so I dare to execute the plan. Our house has stairs into everything, so I carry her to the front door and remind her that I did that when we came home from our honeymoon. She grins.

I place her on the couch. She rubs her hand on it and says, "Mine."

I say, "Yes, you picked it out."

She grins, feels it more, and listens to the music I have playing. Later, I wheel her around the rest of the house. We go into each room. Much of it is sparse as we moved out, then I moved back into the garage last August (looong story). She recognizes things and enjoys herself.

I wheel her to the table where I set out some veggies and fruit with a bowl of grapes nearby. I turn away to grab something and turn back. She is reaching into the bowl grabbing a few grapes and eating them...like one at a time and chewing and everything. This is a BIG DEAL. She has not initiated an action like that in months.

Later, I wheel her out on the deck. We have lots of trees. She looks up at them and smiles. She leans forward and asks me to rub her back. Again, BIG DEAL. She does not look up much and does not ask for things like that. Being a smitten husband, I oblige.

I take her back to the dining room for some light dinner. It was nothing fancy, some chicken and dumplings. I give her a small portion, because, you know...her. I bring the first spoon up, and she says, "Here," and takes the spoon from my hand and starts using it. She is spooning her food, bringing it to her mouth, not spilling anything, and not picking at her food, but eating voraciously. Who stole my wife and replaced her with my wife?!

She finishes her dinner while my mouth is on the floor. I cannot form sentences. I am in shock. I think I mutter, "Are you still hungry?" She says, "Yeah."

I hand her mine. She eats much of that the same way— other than me holding the dish, completely unassisted!

I sit in awe.

After a few minutes she says, "...have to go." I inquire where. "Go back." After multiple clarifications, it was clear she meant back to the facility.

I ask, "Did you have a nice time?"

She paused for just a moment, "Yeah...great."

I ask, "Do you like me?"

She looks up and smiles, "Yeah. I love you."

"But you want to go now?"

"Yeah...go back. They should go."

I place her in the car and drive her back rather than forcing the overnight. I take her to her room and lay her down. She repeats, "That was just, just, just...wonderful."

I ask if she wants to go back to the house again someday. She says, "Yeah...anytime."

WHAT?!?!? How is she having this conversation?

She then puckers for me to kiss her. Of course, I oblige. Again, HUGE DEAL. She has not initiated a kiss in like two years. I have to ask for them and then do not always get one. This is the same woman that will often say ten words in two days and rarely carries on a clear conversation.

I turn on the Beach Boys. A caregiver tells Maureen she will come by soon to help her into her pajamas. She just smiles contently lying there. I...I don't' know, but I think I just had a really great date night. I am left with a happy heart.

We had a couple of great days. You savor them when you can. I jumped the gun and tried bringing her back to the house the next day. That moment we pulled into the drive, she saw the house and said, "No, no, no."

I explained, "It's our home baby."

"No. They, they, no."

She got very flustered, so I turned the car around, and we drove back to the facility. I likely pushed for too much too close together.

That next day went back to just a ten-word day, so we sat in silence holding hands and enjoying the sun and the courtyard. What I would have given to know if past memories just like that quiet one we had right then could still run through her mind. We had some memorable and peaceful times together. I thought I would wait a few weeks before trying another major outing.

FTD runs hot and cold. You have good times and not so good. These shifts could happen even multiple times in a single day.

AFTD Social Media Post – 8/29/19

WEARY BUT WORTH IT

FTD is a thief, plain and simple. FTD has robbed me of the ability to look to the future or to have hope. Wonderful experiences are often met with the opposite, minutes or hours later: it is FTD's cruel joke.

Well I stole something back from FTD—the ability to appreciate the moment. That is mine. I do not know what will come next, but I accept that. I count on nothing. I live and love her in the moment. Creating that mindset is exhausting sure, but so worth it.

Today:

Visit 1 (8:15 a.m.–9:30 a.m.): I stop by as a pre-visit before her mother. She was dressed and being helped with breakfast. I gave her one of my smiles and "Ta-Das". She looks up sternly and asks, "What?" I have learned to freeze this for a three-count. She suddenly smiles (recognition) and says, "Oh, good." After a hug and kiss, I switch with the caregiver to continue feeding her. Cereal is ok, but she likes fruit better. I get her to drink the Ensure. She is chatty and happy to see me. She strokes my arm and pats my cheek and the top of my head. Others would think it clumsy, but for me, bliss. I say I am going to bring her mother. I kiss her and tell her I will be right back and let the staff know.

Visit 2 (10:15 a.m.–11:30 a.m.): With her mother, I return. I find her still in the grand room but withdrawn. I try the "Ta-Da" again, but only get a slight response. She looks through her mother. There is the noise of their TV, people, etc. I move her to a quieter part of the facility for the three of us. I lift her from Geri chair to couch. She talks a little, nothing making sense. She was generally accusatory toward her mother, me, and random other passersby. For one hour, a lot of looking down and being sullen and silent. We take her to a table for her lunch. I tell her I love her and will be back. I drop off her mother.

Visit 3 (2:30 p.m.–4:00 p.m.): Just a "quick stop" to see if her spirits are better. She is on her bed compulsively folding a blanket. With my same "Ta-Da", she smiles big, "Oh great. Now we, we, we...have some fun. I've been looking for him, him, you." Hmm—I planned on a little visit, but better ramp it up. I offer a quick outing to her favorite, Starbucks. She fires back, "Let's go go." On with her socks and shoes, out the door and lifting her into the car. She says, "Oh, you, you did that so nice." With frappuccino and fruit/cheese box and a close-by park, there is music, drinking, eating, and talking (no sense of the story but joyful).

Soon the talk stops, she looks distant, no longer eating or drinking. After a failed bit of coaxing, I take her back to the facility and the grand room. I must run some errands, so I tell her I love her and will be back.

Visit 4 (6:00 p.m.–7:30 p.m.): At the same table after some dinner, she looks pale and completely out of it. The "Ta-Da" had zero effect. She feels hot. I return her to her room and help staff get her changed and ready for bed. She is generally agitated. They leave, and I dim the lights. Curled on her side in a fetal position, I pull just a sheet over her. We stare at each other. I tell her I will love her the rest of my life.

She stutters back, "I live live live live love love love love too. (Pause) I am so scared." I ease her fears best I can. She grips my hand hard. I choose not to do music but let her spend several moments drifting off.

When I think she is asleep, I stand to leave, and she opens her eyes and looks at me. I caress her forehead and tell her to, "Sleep well, good night, I love you."

She says emphatically, "We are us."

"We are baby. Nobody else, just us, you and me." I say softly.

She says yeah and lets out a contented sigh. I wipe my tear, kiss her again on the forehead, and this time she stays asleep. I leave.

I write this tonight, completely emotionally spent. I am weary, but love with my wife is always worth being weary for. I will see her again in the morning.

Yes, FTD left me weary, but its impact went beyond just Maureen and I, it also loomed over our finances. With the savings completely gone for a couple of months now, we also had growing debt that I could still manage for now. With the care facility, caregiving costs, the mortgage, and necessities, we lived each month just a little beyond our means.

I could put the house back on the market with a different realtor but had little hope it would sell this time of year. As we approached the fall, I knew the site would not show as well as in the spring. Bigger families that might want such a large house had already made their moves for the year.

I started selling some household items of no emotional value for me or her kids.

We had some bonds that I sold.

I cut absolutely all unnecessary expenses (except for her weekly flowers).

With a few calls, I determined I could get a home equity loan if necessary but waited to pull that trigger. I built up my confidence that we could make it to next summer, but the house would have to sell by then or I'd have to take out the loan. I would have to take less for the house, just to get it gone. I thought come the spring, we would list it for a great price. We knew what others sold for, and we would undercut those. Even if it still left us with some debt, we could manage it better than the mortgage now and avoid falling into a deeper hole. I had a plan.

AFTD Social Media Post – 9/8/19

GRATEFUL DESPITE THE STORMS

We know the phrase, "a storm is coming." On this site, we all know the storm is here, been here, and is not leaving anytime soon. We do workarounds to get through it and find small ways to celebrate. To just hunker down and wait for it to pass...no, that does not work. I think this group is the premier authority on "making the best of it."

I think back to Maureen telling me how she used to love the thunderstorms where she grew up in Redmond, Oregon. For those unaware, Redmond is in Central Oregon, about two and a half hours from Portland and up on the High Desert. Maureen lived next to a canyon, so the thunderstorms were particularly loud and exciting. She loved to watch them.

As an adult, she says she has no desire to live in Redmond again, for a variety of reasons, but she still loves a good storm. We had a thunderstorm here several days ago, but yesterday was just a light one. I took her outside last night under the protection of a gazebo.

I held her hand as she listened and felt it around her. It had been a quiet tempest of a day.

She has spoken almost no words for the last two days. She has barely cracked a smile. Yesterday she was more self-isolating than normal. While I tried to coax words and smiles out of her, she has not wanted "to play". That is ok. I move to Plan B and just spend the time with her. She will still hold my hand anytime I reach for hers, so I cherish that.

Her cancer wounds have been worse the last few days. They are not bigger, just oozing more and more discolored.

They clean it and rebandage, but little can be done. Hospice has been great. She has had a few moments where she felt pain, and we got that under control. It is quiet rain in our lives.

She has been sleeping more, so I go get some tea. I have been reading Marala Scott's With Gratitude. I welcome the warm drink, good book, and rain.

Her mood could be the change to fall. The days are getting shorter and cooler. She often gets melancholy this time of year. Perhaps FTD does not change that.

I did change the décor on her door and in her room to autumn but tried to make it festive with bright colors. I change it up every month. Some things remain consistent, and other things change to help her understand the passing seasons. I taped brightly colored, falling leaves to her door. There are three wandering male residents very taken by this, and in a day, I have seen a few removed. They may not make it the weekend. I have no worries: it is just part of a care facility, like rain's pitter patter.

Speaking of, yesterday, I take her to her room for a midday nap, and the door had been left unlocked. We try to keep it locked due to wanderers. One of the men was in there and peed himself and all over the floor. I left Maureen out of the room and politely asked the man to, "Please come out. This isn't your room."

"I peed," he explained.

"Yes. I can see that. Let us get you taken care of." I then call for a caregiver down the hall, and they jump into re-action and tend to him and strip everything in her room and thoroughly clean the whole room top to bottom. Our thunder rolls through.

I take Maureen to one of the sitting areas, and we lean our heads together and listen to soft music and drown out the rain.

Last night, she was sleepy after the gazebo, so I got her into her pajamas and carried her to her bed. She grabbed my neck a little tighter than normal. It felt good. I got her tucked in. While I gave her a hug, unsolicited, she kissed me on the cheek. She said no words, but she said every-thing. Yeah, we talk our own language even when we say no words.

"Life isn't about waiting for the storm to pass. It's about learning how to dance in the rain." —Vivian Greene

I am grateful I have a twenty-five-second video from about eighteen months ago of us dancing. We were in our kitchen but in the middle of the storm.

Several times between when I thought I would lose her that prior December to nine months later, she kept rallying. She started eating more. She even grabbed the utensil herself a few times and worked at using it.

She remained in good spirits during most of my visits. She even laughed a bit in her sleep. She continued to recognize my voice as I came into the room even though she had her eyes shut.

Not to say she did not still relapse during that time too, but I saw a general stability and spirit in her. Some nights when I tucked her into bed and told her I loved her, she offered that reciprocating language and said, "I love you so, so, so totally." I liked that.

However, I worked; I had to. As such, I could not stay with her all the time. I relied on caregiving staff to keep this newfound momen-tum going. They no doubt had some great caregivers and med-aids, but you do not get to pick who you get, so the high turnover in those positions would often leave you with the new batch that had to get trained all over again.

The facility had undeniably become a godsend that last year for us. I knew that they tried hard most of the time. I just expected more for the money that we kept spending. I expected better training. They often got more focused on their duties rather than how to properly engage each resident. Again, great people, poor system.

Part of Maureen's better spirits may have included physical relief too. We had secured an alternate mattress for Maureen a few weeks back. While the bed frame allowed us to change her angle at the head, waist, and knees, this mattress allowed us to also adjust the firmness so as to take the pressure off her joints.

Additionally, I found three orthopedic pillows online for her to sit on in the Geri chair and the wheelchair (with a spare). These would take the pressure off her tailbone due to her weight loss.

We made strides, and she showed some spirit. I had missed that fire in her.

Scott's Journal – 9/14/19

What can I do to improve what I am doing for Maureen?

What does she love? She loves music. I play it for her all the time, but how can I improve her quality of life through music?

She separated herself from her piano playing a couple years back. The FTD just made it too hard for her to initiate activity and to play notes. She spent her whole childhood being told when she hit a wrong note: she probably has a natural aversion to it now. She does not get that it does not matter, just do what you enjoy.

Her facility has an old keyboard that they keep in a corner with the lid closed except for church on Sundays. In my stroll with Maureen today she was alert, so I pulled it out. I put back the lid, turned it on, and rolled her up to it. Do not ask permission, beg forgiveness. I sat beside her.

I played a few notes. She said, "That sounds wonderful." I asked her to touch the keys. She could not tell her hands to do it. She just stared at the keyboard. I played and offered again—nothing. I took her hand and held it as I played, like she was playing. I removed my hand and left her fingers on the keys. She took a long time and felt the keys but did not know how to press them. I showed her again with my hand on hers. I removed it again and asked her to play a note. Her fingers rested and moved back and forth, then landed on one note—Middle C. I congratulated her, but she pulled her hand back. I said, "You can play more if you want."

"No. Not now," she said. I did not push.

I am encouraged this afternoon, so I reached out to a local music therapist. We spoke for forty-five minutes about how they might engage Maureen. I got to tell one more person about FTD. I spoke about the moments today, her background, condition, etc. They are going to come and assess and work up a plan of how to simply engage her to her comfort level. They have several handheld instruments that take almost no effort to make a sound—just shake, bang, or blow.

I have no idea what to expect. Yes, it costs money, but as music has been such a large part of her life, I think I owe it to her to step up my game.

I thought maybe the piano felt too daunting. I also needed to remind myself that we cannot go back, only forward. I had to reframe (to borrow a therapy term) my thinking not to try and restore or recreate the past but to create new joys out of what we find available in the present. While she played the piano before, maybe now she could simply make sounds with simpler objects. All the studies I had read told me we should try.

I saw her happier right now. I wanted to celebrate that and try to find ways to enrich her life rather than giving in to FTD. I thought I would try again at a trip to our favorite beach. I thought just for one night. She loved the beach.

AFTD Social Media Post – 9/21/19

CHANGING THE TRAGEDY NARRATIVE

I am so very smitten with my wife. No, it goes deeper than that...much deeper.

I am borrowing this title from a breadth of work in the last two years I believe first coined by Bill Thomas, a geriatrician, and then a study by Lois Holzman and workshops by Dr. Susan Massad and Mary Fridley, "The Joy of Dementia ('You've got to be kidding)".

They note that we often try to correct dementia behavior back to our perception of normal, which can cause frustration on everyone's part. While things certainly do become more difficult as dementia progresses, the more we adapt, flex, and expand our ideas of how things are supposed to be, we might just create some of the joy we are looking for.

As many of you know, a post I shared a couple months back of me trying to make a moment for my wife with a trip to the beach got cut short. Her pain meds gave her motion sickness. I will spare you the reliving of the details. With an anti-nausea patch in place, we tried again this week with great success.

My wife has always loved the beach, and Cannon Beach is her favorite. We Oregonians take our beaches with a level of wind, rain, and lukewarm temperatures because we are tough, and we know that seventeen minutes of sunshine will soon come. As it turned out, our trip had no rain, almost no wind, and mild to warm temperatures. It was a perfect stay.

Part of the adaptation is removing her triggers: dense population, hurried schedules, and busyness. I brought her out Thursday midday and returned her Friday midday. I checked into the hotel Wednesday and out on Saturday. It involved a lot of driving back and forth on my part but took schedule and check-in/check-out activities off her plate. I focused on simple fun.

Our fun was a beautiful room with a gorgeous panoramic view of the beach; light in-room foods that I had brought based on her current preferences; rest; a beach entry that was wheelchair accessible; quiet time sitting on the sand bundled and staring at the setting sun; ice cream and a roll in front of familiar shops; returning to our room a little after seven to prepare for an early retirement and sleep together (which we had not done in months); waking in the morning slowly at her pace; staring at the beach a little more over a modest breakfast in-room; returning to her facility with rest immediately following.

There were smiles, kisses, comments about it being "nice" and "beautiful", and some intent studying of the waves. The singular purpose of the trip was her joy. Did she feel joy? Yes. Little things that happened and did not happen tell me so.

I chose NOT to go down memory lane with her but instead make this trip about her present joy. In a vaguely familiar setting, I hoped that it might be easier for her to achieve.

This morning though as I checked out alone (after returning her to her facility yesterday afternoon), I strolled the six-ish blocks of old town. It was our favorite part. The first rain of the trip started and spritzed my head, reminding me of years not so long ago.

Yuletides sells Christmas decor 365 days. The Bronze Coast Gallery broke our pocketbook more than once with amazing art. The Driftwood w/outdoor seating and firebox was a fave dinner spot, but if cooler temps prevailed, we would head into Morris's Fireside or grab a slice of pizza at Pizza a'fetta, always followed by a Schwietert's cone and candy for our ice cream (like this trip).

In the mornings, if Maureen were feeling sleepy, I would go get coffee and bagels at any number of shops and bring it back to the room where she was wrapped in a blanket. If we were early to rise, a walk on the sand followed by the Cannon Beach Bakery when it opened at seven.

Tee Har's was great for her Life is Good clothing or La Luna Loca for her bohemian side. Archimedes Gallery was a newer find with art that appealed to Maureen. Geppetto's Toy Shoppe was great for gifts when the grandkids were small.

Sometimes though, we would just window shop at realtors for a beach house "someday" or go into Steidel's Art and watch him draw Mallory Mouse in a house looking itself like out of someone's imagination.

Alone with my thoughts and the drizzle of the rain, I was tempted to be sad because she does not feel that old joy from before. However, that is focusing on the "tragedy narrative". We made a new memory this week, and that is our new joy.

That post captured the wonderful moments and stopped just before the anxiety.

That Saturday morning, I had packed and checked out early, but stayed to have some breakfast and walk the streets and potentially check out the art festival. At 10:40, though, I got a call that Maureen had started seizure-like symptoms and that they had given her half of an Ativan to try and stop them. It had not yet started working. During the course of the three-minute call, I briskly walked/ran back to the car, started it, and pulled out of town. My heart raced, rising though my chest. I was panicking. Everything seemed like she would die, me not with her, ninety minutes away. She seemed so good last night.

I hung up and drove, frustrated at the traffic in front of me. I could not get around them 'till the passing lanes. Several troopers monitored the highway too, and I could not afford to get stopped. She cannot die now, I thought. She cannot die feeling alone without me.

I got back to her care facility around 12:10—no gas, car just on fumes, but it got me there.

I found her sleeping (thank God) with a second half of Ativan. She had not had Ativan before, so it really wiped her out. Shortly after I arrived, a nurse from hospice also got to the facility. All Maureen's vitals read fine and within good margins. I stayed with her a couple of hours and only left when they told me they saw no imminent threat, knowing I could get there from our house in just ten minutes.

With a deep breath, I went home and unpacked. I took care of a few things and then headed back over. The events had left me emotionally spent. Back in her room, I saw her still resting with her eyes closed. I told her I loved her many times, and she would grin slightly and pucker. Due to her rolled over posture in bed, I could not easily get my lips to hers, so I put a finger to her lips. She kissed my finger several times. She seemed ok.

I left to grab a bite and then returned. She now looked a little more lucid—still dazed but awake. I turned her from her side to her back and raised her head, wanting to get fluids in her and perhaps a few bites, given how frail she looked.

During the whole time with her that day and the next, she did not have the more violent shaking they described to me that first morning. She would, however, every three to four minutes, almost go rigid and grab the mattress firmly. She behaved like she was on some sort of a vertigo trip—like falling or a sudden jolt. Sometimes she smiled and giggled lightly and other times her eyes went wide with surprise. I wondered if she had a reaction to the medicine.

I told her I loved her, and she said she loved me too. I thought, "We can get through this." However, it made me aware that, emotionally, I had not "readied" myself at all for her to die. I found it all too hard.

I also came to realize that life does not care if you get "ready". It does not care if you think it all too hard.

AFTD Social Media Post – 10/6/19

CLINGING

I have tried this last year to bring optimism, love, humor, perspective, and hopefully some joy to this courageous group. I often ask us all to find that little sliver of joy in a day and to celebrate the magnificence of the ordinary. Some days it has been hard. This last two weeks has been among the hardest.

I am reminded of Morgan Harper Nichols, a young writer and singer that is wise beyond her years. "Cling to joy. Audacious, unbridled joy, that looks for light in everything. Even while you're waiting."

The tee-up this last two weeks has been her sudden seizure-like shaking on a day with me ninety minutes away and my heart pounding out of my chest. This has been followed by her eating even less, stomach always queasy, losing more weight than I thought possible, liquid stool coming from her cancer wound, elevated pulse, visibly isolating herself, and hospice telling me last Thursday morning, "this is looking like the end."

As I have stated many times, the love I bear for my wife is immeasurable. I am both prepared and completely unprepared. For two weeks up to this moment has included my clearing of work meetings and increased presence at her side, helping anyway I can with her comfort, and trying food or drink for her any time of the day or night.

As I drove back to visit with her tonight, I did that thing that maybe just men do when we fight back tears. It is where you tighten your whole face and pull up the skin to either side of your nose as though you smelled something particularly foul just to control a sob.

You squint your eyes tight to hold back tears, when all you really do is wring your eyes out, and the tears flow anyway. You start that low wail that you try to hold back by constricting your throat, which just makes it sound even more like anguish. And your nose runs like a faucet, and, counter to decorum, you just do not care.

Shift focus: Joy—Joy—Joy:

I received a good kiss from her four or five days ago.

I have a job with flexibility.

In response to me telling her I love her, she did offer a week ago, "I I I love love much."

I look hard for that joy-like pinpoints of daylight in a dark forest.

I get there tonight and greet her as I do, but no real response. I hold her hand at her bedside for quite some time. I make that same face again and everything running all over but bite my lip to keep back the wail and not fluster her. Such a profound feeling of "missing her" washes over me.

I receive a couple words from her here and there. Her eyes remain closed, in a daze, no sense, no purpose known to me, just meant FOR me. I receive the words and agree with their hidden message, as that is what I do. I lean down and ask for a kiss. It is so very faint as though the muscles are just too strained, but it is there.

I brush her hair from her face and my tears from her skin and sit quietly holding her hand with both of mine. She squeezes back. That is some joy.

I am not sure who is clinging more, she or I. It is probably both of us.

I told Maureen's mother what hospice said the same day that they told me. I think we had so many prior "this is it's" that it did not make an impression on her. I remember her reaction well, "Thanks for letting me know."

I told her kids, who visited the prior weekends. They just saw her very sleepy, and she may have not even understood her kids had visited. Her son said he would try and come that next Saturday the 12th.

I hardly left her side that week.

Earlier in the week, she had gotten a little agitated, and I had calmed her with light touches back and forth across her arms and stomach. I found even holding her hand seemed calming for her, like she knew my personal touch. Her eyes were seemingly always closed.

It seemed that she often wanted to say something but simply could not. So, I reminded her of happier times—telling her stories of our adventures together like riding bikes down ancient roads outside of Beaune, France with short stone walls between towns only built for the wine they produced, or how cliff divers caught us by surprise on the coast of Mazatlan and how we danced for hours later that night at the Day of the Dead Festival, much like our dancing to the Cajun music of New Orleans during Mardi Gras or to the classic rock on New Year's Eve on the luxury yacht, The Portland Spirit, back home.

I also reminded her of how many people loved her. I would get very light, content, but wandering "Mm-hmms."

I also told her through my tears that she could just let go if she wanted. I told her she did not need to hang on anymore and that God had a happy place for her to dance.

I went to the facility on Wednesday, October 9th in the mid-afternoon. Maureen was sitting in the dining area of the grand room. I walked up to her and kneeled on the floor. Her head was slung down, and her eyes mostly closed. I caressed her arm and gently said, "Ta Da." She gave me a grin, so I knew she knew. I kissed her on the cheek and held her hand. She squeezed back.

I asked the caregiver sitting next to her if she had eaten or drank anything. "No," she said. "A little this morning." So frail.

I leaned in to offer a quiet, "I love you" and another kiss.

I tried to get her to eat or drink a little. Other than a couple of sips of water with her straw, nothing. Her eyes remained almost shut.

I wheeled her into her room, and though barely 4:00 p.m., suggested we get her in her pajamas. Maureen only reacted slightly. I kept giving her assurances as I dressed her in her pajamas—her favorite blue flannel ones. I knew she liked the soft feel against her skin. She never struggled. I lay her on her bed, tucked her in, and elevated her head.

I decided to stay the night. Things did not seem right. SHE did not seem right. I saw her fading before my eyes.

One of the staff gave me a blanket and pillow. I returned to her room. Maureen lay there so still, so frail, so quiet.

I sat beside her bed, holding her hand, speaking softly to her with simple, quiet words of love. I did not know what else to do. Through the tears, I told her that if she wanted to let go, I understood. I told her she would find peace. I lied to her and told her that I would find peace too. I leaned toward her and gave her a light hug with my cheek across her face. She puckered and lightly kissed my cheek. I said, "I love you," and kissed her lips, and those lips kissed me back ever so gently, like leaves that would blow apart in the slightest breeze.

I held her hand for hours. I played just a few of her songs. She made some noises as though humming along or even a light singing. I kept talking softly to her and occasionally leaned over to hug her again, to get those same gentle wisps of lips pecking me back on the cheek. Nothing in my life had ever felt so tender, so loving, and at the same time so sad.

I did not know what to do. As I said before, we had gotten baptized together some twenty-two years prior. She had a good soul. She had a strong Christian faith. With a one-handed search (never letting go of hers), I found a passage for the dying on my phone. I was looking not so much for a last rite but just something I thought would sound like the right thing to her. I knew I wasn't a priest, just a man wholly and completely in love with his wife and wanting to do anything, everything for her. I read to her softly:

Prayers for the Dying

Dear Heavenly Father, with heavy hearts we come to You. You are Almighty Creator God, holy and full of grace and love. Our hearts are heavy because of a life that is leaving us. Death engulfs us Lord. Fear is waiting to take us down. Thank You Father, that because of Jesus, You know our pain and sorrow intimately. Thank You that Jesus knows the way through this dark shadow. Take the hand of our dear sister and make Yourself known. Guard our hearts and minds in Christ Jesus. Keep that which is Your own and take it into eternity to be with You. In Jesus, death is but a shadow. Jesus has swallowed up its sorrows and pain. Thank You Jesus for the cross. Thank You Jesus for the resurrection. Lord, we are before You, confessing that You are Lord of all, the gatekeeper to eternal life. Your grace and love abound even as our sin seems ever increasing. Take our hands Lord and lead us through. We lay our fears at your feet. Your promise is that You —and You alone— will come to take us home. As it says in Psalm 23:4:"Even though I walk through the valley of the shadow of death, I will fear no evil, for you are with me; your rod and your staff, they comfort me."

Thank you for the comfort we find in Your presence. Through the Holy Spirit we know Your presence is with us. Send us Your peace Lord; the peace that passes all understanding. Do not let us waiver and doubt. Give us a faith that is ever-lasting. We release our lives into Your hands. As we wait and watch, we know Lord that none of us will escape this journey through death. Teach us how to embrace it with faith. Give us strength to hold up those who are stepping closer to seeing You face to face. Take away the fear in the heart of our loved one who will soon see You; let them find peace in Your grace, comfort in Your love, and strength in Your mighty power over death. Comfort us as our grief seems to overpower us.

You are a good, just, righteous, and loving Father. Do not let us grow bitter in this shadow of death. But pierce our hearts with a joy that we cannot fathom or understand. A joy that is above all that is corrupted here on earth. Jesus, you wept over death and so too we weep. But it is a grief and a mourning that holds joy on the other side. You are conqueror of all; and so, we trust You. We trust that You will do what is right, what is loving. Whether in death or in life Your will is accomplished, and You are sovereign. May we know Your presence, Lord. Keep us ever aware of Your

loving hand guiding us through all things. In the name of
Jesus, we pray, Amen.

I asked God to receive her and asked Maureen softly that if she could, to please save a seat for me so I could see her again someday... and a dance for me so I could hold her again. I let out silent tears and a lot of pain.

I held her hand all night. To have a chance of sleep, I lay in her Geri chair and she in her bed. I lined us head to toe so we could look at each other (though her eyes were just slits) and hold hands the whole night, even if we dozed off. I refused to let her feel alone, even for a moment.

Other than a few head bobs, I did not sleep. I held her hand for hours—occasionally playing soothing music including her "Calling on Angels" and "I Can Only Imagine."

Her breathing seemed normal and a regular rhythm. I watched her chest rise and fall throughout the night as I sat holding her hand.

About 4 a.m., I moved back to a regular chair and still held her hand—professing my eternal love for her in a soft and calming voice. I assured her she would not pass alone, that she would find peace, as would I (it still felt like lying).

I never let go of her hand that morning, just silently crying for what I saw unfolding. She responded only with slight squeezes of my hand.

As I said, I had watched her chest rise and fall for hours and listened to her breath—neither strained nor wet, just soft and steady. A couple of minutes before six that morning, I saw her chest rise and fall more slowly, perhaps taking twice as long as before. Again, not strained breathing, simply slowing, her chin rising slightly with the breath, then slower yet, then it stopped. Mine did too.

I did not let go; would not. I held her hand for a couple of minutes to make sure of what I had seen. I waited. Nothing. With one hand, I called the med-aid on duty, Gina, and asked her to come in.

Gina came promptly but calmly. Sitting beside Maureen's bed with both hands holding hers and tears running down my face, I said in my calmest voice, "I think she's passed. Can you check for me?" She did as I asked. "You're right honey, she passed. I'm so sorry Scott."

She placed her hand on my shoulder and held back her own tears. I wailed softly at first.

"Is there anything that I can do?" she asked.

"I guess we're supposed to call hospice. I think…" and I trailed off, not able to think.

Gina left and closed the door behind her. I wailed again, but louder, alternating kisses between her hand and her lips and her cheeks and her forehead. I wet her with my tears. I felt lost. The room had one dim light on. I sat there at the bedside with the love of my life, holding her hand, and kissing it and saying things to her, professions of love that I do not recall now.

Maybe an hour later, a person from hospice interrupted our time. I had not met this person before. At least, I did not think so. I really did not even look up. Gina came back in too. They offered those words of encouragement when one does not know what else to say. I both heard them and did not—I was in no state to receive them with any understanding anyway. I kept holding her hand, clinging.

The hospice worker knew she had to target her questions to get me directed. "Do you have someone in mind to come take her?" So detached.

"Mt. Scott Funeral Home is nearby. She had an aunt and uncle with services there." I honestly do not know how I came up with that name amid my agonizing grief. I think because the first wave had passed, and the next wave had not yet hit. She said she would take care of it and left. Before Gina left, she said, "Scott. You are not going to want to be here when they lift her and cover her up. It is too hard. One of us can help." She closed the door behind her.

Alone again with my baby. I had never let go of her hand. I had not interlaced our fingers as much as held her whole hand. My whole heart and life washed over me. I kept her hand warm in mine—just like she liked it. I kissed her lips again. I kissed her forehead again. Her forehead had started to cool. "Of course," I thought and wailed again.

Her death did not, I think, feel totally real for me yet. I sat there holding her hand after all. She still lay here right next to me. I had never witnessed death firsthand. Relatives and friends had died but someone just called you, and you went to a service. Yes, close and dear people but not...her—not the most important person in the world to me. I did not watch them pass like I had just witnessed here.

My mind started racing as to whether I did everything right for her. Should I do something else right now? No, just sit in the moment, just hold her hand for these last moments. I brushed some of my tears from her cheek and brushed that same hand along her hair—the hair I would never get to brush again.

I talked to her softly. The tears ran dry on my cheeks now. I kissed her again on the forehead, cooler still. I sat my vigil at her bedside. I just stared at my beautiful wife, here yet gone.

I think sometime after 8:00 that morning, the funeral home tech arrived. They opened the door and the lone tech introduced herself. Please do not ask me to tell you her name. Following her were Gina and the kind young lady, Taylor, from the front desk, and I think maybe the Director, though I honestly cannot remember. Taylor entered crying. She had started working there the same week that I brought Maureen to this facility.

With everyone there, I finally lay Maureen's hand down gently on her stomach, whispered something soft to her, and then stood and turned to Taylor, who outstretched her arms for a hug and told me how very sorry she felt. We both cried briefly on each other's shoulders.

The funeral home tech confirmed Maureen's passing, something Gina had done hours earlier.

Only then did I really take in what she had brought with her. She had a gurney. On it lay a velvet bag that she opened, revealing a small sheet, a half quilt, a plastic bag, and a small tag. The only people in the room now were me, the tech, Gina, and my Maureen.

The tech lay the sheet over Maureen's torso and explained that she had to put the tag on Maureen's ankle (Oh God, I see it really happening). The tech then said, "We have to lift her onto the gurney." The velvet bag lay splayed with the plastic bag inside. Gina asked, "Scott, do you want me to help her?"

I said softly, "No. This is mine to do."

I lifted Maureen's head and torso with her hands on her stomach, and the tech lifted her legs, and we placed my baby on the gurney. She began to lap the plastic over her legs and torso with me standing there staring. I held Maureen's head gently in both my hands, leaned down, and kissed her forehead so very intentionally and lovingly, as though my kiss could still somehow bring her back. With tears flowing, I whispered, "Goodbye my baby."

The tech asked if I needed more time. I said no. She asked if I wanted her taken out with her head not yet covered. I said no. She lapped the bag and zipped it. She held the quilt and asked if Maureen had served in the military. I said no. She turned the flag upside down and the flower side up and placed it over the velvet bag with my beloved wife inside. She asked If I wanted to follow her out. I said no.

They wheeled her out and closed the door and left me with just the one dim light on.

My knees collapsed, dropping me to her bed.

No, no, no, no.

I sat alone in that small, empty room for a long time…and wept.

AFTD Social Media Post – 10/10/19 (late that evening)

Today, I am saddened far more than I have ever been, but also hopeful that she is dancing now, dancing somewhere beautiful…

Maureen Patrick-Rose was born April 27, 1950 and lived joyously to October 10, 2019

> "Day by day and night by night we were together—all else has long been forgotten by me,
>
> I remember I say only that woman who passionately clung to me,
>
> Again we wander, we love, we separate again,
>
> Again she holds me by the hand, I must not go,
>
> I see her close beside me with silent lips sad and tremulous."
>
> —Walt Whitman

I will be back to this AFTD family soon—I just need a little time. Thank you for all you do and have done for me.

THE END

Conclusion

*F*TD devastates families. Caring for the needs of your loved one continues well after their passing. Grieving lasts even longer. Nobody can tell you how to do it, though they try. A lesson I keep trying to learn: let others help me more. I took, and take, a lot of walks. I remember with smiles and tears.

I held Maureen's service on Sunday, November 3, 2019, just a few weeks after her passing. I took care of all the details to keep myself busy—a project manager and all. I had moments alone of overwhelming grief that required I stop and take it all in. Sometimes I just collapsed on the floor in a heap of screams, tears, and weariness. Afterward, I stood myself up and forged ahead, reminding myself to honor her well.

After the day-of calls to her kids and mother, I let them know frequently what I had planned so they could comment if they felt the need or desire. I shared the photos I selected for her tribute with them, and they added a few. I made all the painful calls to the closest friends and family myself and shared a lot of tears. Venue, flowers, catering, obits, announcements, music, tributes, and on and on. These mini projects helped me manage the grief and focus on doing the best for her. I always asked, "What would Maureen want?"

The funeral home looked, I am sorry to say, dreadful. I felt convinced if I had held the service there, my beautiful, kind, and understanding wife would have chastised me from beyond. I instead chose a lovely space on an old Victorian home site that many had used for weddings. It held gardens and lots of windows. As luck would have it, the sun shone brightly that day and made it beautiful. Sunlight flooded the room and warmed the heart. Despite a normally cold, damp fall, on this day, the sun kept it dry and warm enough that people ventured outside and took pictures with friends and family they had not seen in a long time. Such things occur at these gatherings.

Many spoke on Maureen's behalf, including of course myself. Two ladies from Parkview Memory Care came to the service. Family from her first husband had also come. People from my work attended. I had hoped at least one person from her work would come, as I had notified Tri-met and posted a notice in the driver break lounge, but no. Perhaps simply too much time had passed.

I looked around at so many friends and family, but also people that had never met Maureen. People from the Pittock Mansion came to show their respects, recognizing us as not just donors, but our romantic attachment to the home—good people. Others that I had met through AFTD also arrived. They had heard the stories of Maureen and seen her pictures and wanted to hear more of her life's story.

I had the good fortune of arranging to have the pastor who had officiated our wedding and our ten-year vow renewal there. He would also officiate over this Celebration of Life. It brought our lives together full circle. Others assured me we had a lovely and happy service. I know I struggled to find any joy that day.

My mother came up to me afterward, never I think fully understanding the choices I had made in my life, but she brought none of that up and offered the comfort that, "Maureen was perfect for you." Yes, I thought back to my marriage proposal to Maureen, down on one knee at our park, "The perfect bride for me."

In the time since Maureen's passing, I have struggled profoundly with grief. Mustering motivation each day proves hard. I cry a lot. I remember better times and smile, then cry again. I have ventured to our beach several times and walked in lonely silence. I post pictures and mementos all over our house. I play her favorite music again and again and walk the house like when we walked the halls of her facility. However, I do not have her hand to hold, nor can I dance with her anymore, so I cry again.

I spoke with the hospital regarding grief counselors. They offered little. I had a phone interview and an in-person interview. Both asked the state-required, "Are you having suicidal thoughts?" questions. I said no, so they trailed off and gave general advice on eating well and getting outside and rushed me off the phone or scooted me out the door for their 3:00 appointment. Hospice reached out a couple times.

I know that there are many books on handling grief. I read a bit here and there, and I have come to realize that as long as I bring no harm to myself or others, I will simply learn to live with my grief. My grief has no right or wrong way to process it. In the end, I will simply balance that new "grief piece" of my life with the other pieces. I will always have grief as a part of me, but hopefully not the suffering.

I received many well-wishes and condolences in the weeks that passed:

> "At least she's free now."
> "She wouldn't want you to be sad."
> "She would want you to live your life."
> "You will have a new life."
> "You'll get through this."
> "I'm here for you if you need something."

All well intentioned, all from good people, and all feel worthless most of the time. Again, it comes down to just living with it. I let the tears flow and even watch old movies, read old letters, and look at old pictures that I know will make me cry. I embrace that and let it out.

We do live on with our grief. We also need to carry on. Specific to our situation, I, and many others, have found that FTD can leave your health in ruin:

Physically
Mentally
Spiritually
Relationally
Vocationally
Financially

You have got to climb out, and as long as it takes to get into those situations, it may take even longer to get out. An AFTD friend of mine, ten years younger and also with a wife with FTD, calls it the two-twenty-year recovery. I agree and understand.

Where do you find yourself in your own life? Did your loved one die with you still in your thirties or your fifties? Who passed in your life: your child, spouse, sibling, parent, or friend? With FTD often manifesting as a young onset dementia, it can devastate lives and families. Even striking later in life, what does that do to your retirement planning? Will your physical health have the time to recover? My beloved wife died with me at fifty-two. Recovering my health will take some work. My finances took a huge hit with the savings gone and standing debt. HOWEVER, I would not trade a single moment with her for any of this to go away. We said, "For better or worse," and I love that I had her in my life to commit that promise to.

I placed a note in my home office a month after the service. I gravitate to it most days: "Maureen deserves a legacy that lives well beyond me." That provides the necessary motivation to get me out of bed and to do more, to focus on something greater than my own grief.

I lay her to rest in Eugene, Oregon, near the kids and two hours from me. While I would have preferred having her up in Portland, I wanted her to always have flowers at her site. Up here, I know the kids would rarely make the trek. I know I will trek down frequently. I already have. Someday I too will die, but she will always have kids or grandkids down there, so should always get flowers. She liked flowers.

I encourage you to know your loved one's wishes. Have the hard talks now. Maureen and I walked the memorial park where she now rests. We picked the spot together. Many years earlier, she said she preferred cremation. She said, "Don't you put me in the cold ground in the rain." While I wanted inside the mausoleum, only glass cases remained, and those do not have flower rings.

I went on the exterior wall but under a deep overhang—no rain on you baby. Also, on the outside, I can place (and have placed) flowers at any time of day or night rather than wait for the building to open. I stash a few of the vases in my car and access her site from a side neighborhood. I bring a folding chair, place the flowers, talk to her and read to her, or look at old photos, or write in my journal, or play a song from her playlist, or just sit and look with her at the trees and the mountains and smile and cry. I miss her.

I also look at our old haunts and think about a level of permanence for her and I. I want to capture the love story. She would like that. We have a theater seat in Scappoose and a few scattered pavers in the region. After her passing, I worked with Pittock Mansion, the Portland Parks Department, and the Friends of the Portland

Memory Garden to leave legacies there. I chose simple and understated phrases on benches to remember her and remember us. I periodically leave two anonymous white roses with pink edges at these sites, wrapped in three ribbons: blue "#EndDementia", yellow "Hope", and pink "Forever Love".

I hope these little gestures will cause others to pause in the future and think, "Those two people were very much in love." Maureen would like to cause future smiles.

Our home we built has a bronze plaque:

DESTINY'S HEARTH

A Home of Comfort and Love

Designed by

Maureen and Scott Rose

October 5, 2007

Destiny plays on the meaning of her middle name, LaVaye. Hearth references the kind, loving, simple but elegant way she lived her life and made our house a home. Some future owners will inherit that memory and hopefully honor it.

This book also adds to her legacy. I think it important to not only tell Maureen's story and share this amazing woman with the world, but also to share the steps of her FTD journey so others can learn from it for the sake of their owned loved ones.

Our ongoing battle against FTD by increasing awareness might prove the greatest legacy of Maureen and other loved ones that passed alongside her. This awareness generates passion and resources that lead to research and eventually a cure.

Visit www.theaftd.org to learn more.

AFTD Social Media Post – 4/27/20 (two hundred days after Maureen passed)

THE "LOUD"

My wife's birthday is today. She would have turned seventy. She would have been a youthful seventy if not for the FTD. I will be turning fifty-three this June. That never mattered. It still doesn't. Many people assumed we were the same age, and some even thought that I was older, which made her giggle. She took good care of herself. She ate healthy... mostly. We frequently took long walks and went out dancing. Exercise?! She was not into that "sweaty stuff" as she called it. She liked to swim but only when the temperatures were just right: hence our tropical trips to places like Mexico (she was still a stunner in a swimsuit at sixty-three).

I would have thrown her a surprise party today if not for the FTD. We had a great surprise party on her sixtieth. I invited her closest family and friends (about twenty). They all secretly arrived while I had Maureen out for her Starbucks and her nails. I had it catered with her favorite food and a triple chocolate cake with vanilla ice cream because... well, her favorites. She enjoyed it because it was comfortable. These were people she knew and loved well. It was in the calm of our home and not a loud restaurant.

Maureen had always been a bit of an introvert with people she did not know. Me, I was a bit the opposite. My professional life was...loud. I managed a division of a large company, rallied troops, lead marketing efforts and interviews, and spoke to groups as large as 1,000: all of this without a care.

With Maureen, my personal life could be toned way back. We relished our quiet time together. We did calm, romantic things. Yes, you can find romance even at the farmer's market if you are not afraid to spontaneously dance with your sweetie to the sounds of a street guitarist. She was my balance to the loud. I would still be dancing with her now, if not for the FTD.

I say, "If not for the FTD" because, as you know, it cuts that short. What made her happiest was me adjusting to...well, what made her happiest. FTD changed that weekly, daily, even hourly. That is ok: love makes you nimble. With her FTD, I had to strip away the loud. We would focus on singular, simple things. It's funny that earlier in our relationship, she taught me to appreciate the simpler moments of a sunset or the tide, but now, in FTD, I was teaching her to drown out all the noise and focus on a flower or a photo. FTD made her mind race, so she needed that calm.

We still had joy in that three and a half years of FTD, with simple outings or music or fun foods or one-on-ones with friends or dancing. We still danced. When her condition changed so she paced almost constantly, I broke it up with dance, and she smiled. In her last four to five months when she could not walk, we simply danced differently. We would gaze at each other like we first did almost twenty-three years earlier and sway to a favorite song and leave the loud behind.

Now that FTD has taken her from me, there is a lot of noise to work through. The politics and COVID-19 are everywhere. Work, while I am thankful right now to still have a job, will fill every hour...if I let it. Struggling financials, care for the house, trying not to lose connection with friends and family, and trying to restore my own physical and emotional health is all so very loud. Have you been there? Are you there now?

My balance was taken with Maureen last October. However, surprisingly, I find my grief now helps me with that balance. I should have realized that it would, because Maureen is still with me, intertwined with that grief and drowning out the loud. As I grieve, I cannot hear anything else.

This weekend, I wrapped ribbons around roses that I left anonymously at two spots in town where her modest memorials will go this summer. I also visited her grave with flowers and the same ribbons. I got home, parked the car, stayed still, and cried a bit. I turned on Dylan's "Make You Feel My Love" and closed my eyes. For a moment, I could remember the way she felt leaning against me with my arms around her and us dancing. For three minutes and thirty-two seconds, we drowned out the loud. Happy birthday Maureen. I love you baby.

I honestly do not know how to describe how I feel right now.

I slowly walk, heartbroken by this void but happy that she walked with me for a time.

I would sum up the best experience of my entire life as the collection of all the time that I spent with Maureen. The second best? The time that I now spend grieving. I have the privilege of both.

I do not know where I will travel, but I know she left me a far better person for having walked part of this journey with her. In my grief, I have to figure out what to do with all that she has left behind for me.

She gave me the priceless gifts of her time and love...and we danced.

Maureen said, "We are us."

Yes, we still are baby—forever and one day more.

CPSIA information can be obtained
at www.ICGtesting.com
Printed in the USA
BVHW031941310821
615711BV00007B/57

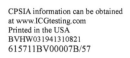

9 781736 820315